W9-AOI-165

Medical Management of Type 2 Diabetes

FOURTH EDITION

Clinical Education Series

Medical Management of Type 2 Diabetes

FOURTH EDITION

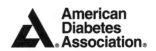

American
Diabetes
Association®

Clinical Education Series

Book Acquisitions	Robert J. Anthony
Project Manager	Laurie Guffey
Production Director	Carolyn R. Segree
Production Coordinator	Peggy M. Rote
Desktop Publishing	Harlowe Typography, Inc.
Design	Wickham & Associates, Inc.

©1998 by the American Diabetes Association, Inc. All Rights Reserved. No part of this publication may be reproduced or transmitted in any form or by any means, electronic or mechanical, including duplication, recording, or any information storage and retrieval system, without the prior written permission of the American Diabetes Association.

Printed in Canada

1 3 5 7 9 10 8 6 4 2

The suggestions and information contained in this publication are generally consistent with the *Clinical Practice Recommendations* and other policies of the American Diabetes Association, but they do not represent the policy or position of the Association or any of its boards or committees. Reasonable steps have been taken to ensure the accuracy of the information presented. However, the American Diabetes Association cannot ensure the safety or efficacy of any product or service described in this publication. Individuals are advised to consult a physician or other appropriate health care professional before undertaking any diet or exercise program or taking any medication referred to in this publication. Professionals must use and apply their own professional judgment, experience, and training and should not rely solely on the information contained in this publication before prescribing any diet, exercise, or medication. The American Diabetes Association—its officers, directors, employees, volunteers, and members—assumes no responsibility or liability for personal or other injury, loss, or damage that may result from the suggestions or information in this publication.

American Diabetes Association
1660 Duke Street
Alexandria, Virginia 22314

Library of Congress Cataloging-in-Publication Data

Medical management of type 2 diabetes.—4th ed.
                           p.   cm. — (Clinical education series)
     Rev. ed. of: Medical management of non-insulin-dependent (type II) diabetes / American Diabetes Association. 3rd ed. c1994.
     Includes bibliographical references and index.
     ISBN 0-945448-93-7 (pbk.)
     1. Non-insulin-dependent   diabetes. I.   American   Diabetes Association. II. Medical   management   of   non-insulin-dependent (type II) diabetes.   III. Series.
     [DNLM: 1. Diabetes Mellitus, Non-Insulin-Dependent.   WK 810 M48791 1998]
RC662.18.M43   1998
  616.4'62—dc21
  DNLM/DLC
  for Library of Congress   98-4107
                                                            CIP

Editorial Advisory Board

EDITOR-IN-CHIEF
David B. Kelley, MD
Olympia, Washington

ASSOCIATE EDITORS
Robert M. Anderson, EdD
Michigan Diabetes Research and
Training Center
The University of Michigan
Medical School
Ann Arbor, Michigan

Janine C. Freeman, RD, CDE
Georgia Center for Diabetes at
Columbia Dunwoody Medical
Center
Atlanta, Georgia

Patti Bazel Geil, MS, RD, CDE
The University of Kentucky
Hospital
Lexington, Kentucky

Marvin E. Levin, MD
Chesterfield, Missouri

**Barbara J. Maschak-Carey,
RNCS, MSN, CDE**
Hospital of the University of
Pennsylvania
Philadelphia, Pennsylvania

David S. Schade, MD
The University of New Mexico
School of Medicine
Albuquerque, New Mexico

MEMBERS
Samuel L. Abbate, MD, CDE
Medcenter One Health Systems
Bismarck, North Dakota

Eva Brzezinski, RD, MS
The University of California at San
Diego Medical Center
San Diego, California

Connie C. Crawley, RD, BS, MS
The University of Georgia
Cooperative Extension Service
Athens, Georgia

John T. Devlin, MD
Maine Medical Center
Portland, Maine

Alan M. Jacobson, MD
Joslin Diabetes Center
Boston, Massachusetts

Lois Jovanovic, MD
Sansum Medical Research
Foundation
Santa Barbara, California

Carolyn Leontos, MS, RD, CDE
The University of Nevada
Cooperative Extension
Las Vegas, Nevada

Peter A. Lodewick, MD
Diabetes Care Center
Birmingham, Alabama

MEMBERS (*Continued*)

Carol E. Malcom, BSN, CDE
Highline Community Hospital
Seattle, Washington

Wylie McNabb, EdD
The University of Chicago Center
    for Medical Education and
    Health Care
Chicago, Illinois

**Virginia Peragallo-Dittko, RN,
    MA, CDE**
Winthrop University Hospital
Mineola, New York

Jacqueline Siegel, RN
St. Joseph Hospital
Seattle, Washington

Tim Wysocki, PhD
Nemours Children's Clinic
Jacksonville, Florida

Contents

A Word about This Guide

The *Medical Management of Type 2 Diabetes* is part of the American Diabetes Association's Clinical Education Series, which also includes *The Health Professional's Guide to Diabetes and Exercise, Medical Management of Type 1 Diabetes, Therapy for Diabetes Mellitus and Related Disorders, Intensive Diabetes Management,* and *Medical Management of Pregnancy Complicated by Diabetes.* The Clinical Education Series was designed to provide health care professionals with the comprehensive information needed to give the best possible medical care to patients with diabetes mellitus.

New information has improved our knowledge about the pathogenesis of diabetes. Although the landmark Diabetes Control and Complications Trial demonstrated the value of glycemic control in patients with type 1 diabetes, many experts believe its findings have implications for the treatment of type 2 diabetes as well. It is clear that proper nutrition, exercise, and excellent blood glucose regulation in addition to attention to blood pressure and lipid levels are key elements in the management of type 2 diabetes. This edition of *Medical Management of Type 2 Diabetes* has been updated to provide state-of-the-art information on these issues, to reflect the most recent clinical practice recommendations from the American Diabetes Association, and to include the new diagnostic and classification criteria adopted by the Association in 1997.

The publication of this book could not have been possible without the expert guidance of many generous contributors and reviewers. The book's focus on pathogenesis, diagnosis and classification, routine management, and maintaining wellness through proper nutrition, exercise, and the treatment of complications was the work of many experts, who laid this comprehensive foundation in the book's previous editions.

The American Diabetes Association believes that you will find this book as useful as its predecessors. Hopefully, it will encourage you to add other American Diabetes Association publications to your library, which can help you manage your patients with diabetes more effectively.

BRUCE R. ZIMMERMAN, MD
Editor-in-Chief
Fourth Edition

PHILIP RASKIN, MD
Editor-in-Chief
Third Edition

HAROLD RIFKIN, MD
HAROLD E. LEBOVITZ, MD
Editors-in-Chief
First and Second Editions

Contributors

EDITOR-IN-CHIEF

Bruce R. Zimmerman, MD
Mayo Clinic
Rochester, Minnesota

CONTRIBUTING EDITORS

Christine A. Beebe, MS, RD, CDE, LD
St. James Hospital and Health Center
Chicago Heights, Illinois

John Buse, MD
University of North Carolina
Chapel Hill, North Carolina

Mayer B. Davidson, MD
Cedars-Sinai Medical Center
Los Angeles, California

David Nathan, MD
Massachusetts General Hospital
Boston, Massachusetts

Matthew C. Riddle, MD
Oregon Health Sciences University
Portland, Oregon

Robert A. Rizza, MD
Mayo Clinic
Rochester, Minnesota

F. John Service, MD, PhD
Mayo Clinic
Rochester, Minnesota

Robert Sherwin, MD
Yale School of Medicine
New Haven, Connecticut

Diagnosis and Classification

Highlights
Diagnosis and Classification

■ Diabetes mellitus is a disorder characterized by hyperglycemia resulting from defects in insulin secretion and/or insulin action. The classification of diabetes mellitus includes four clinical classes: type 1 diabetes, type 2 diabetes, other specific types of diabetes, and gestational diabetes mellitus (GDM). Hyperglycemia not sufficient to meet diagnostic criteria for diabetes is categorized as either impaired fasting glucose (IFG) or impaired glucose tolerance (IGT), depending on whether it is identified on a fasting glucose specimen or after a glucose tolerance test. At least 25% of these patients will eventually have hyperglycemia meeting diagnostic criteria for diabetes.

• Type 1 diabetes was previously called insulin-dependent diabetes mellitus (IDDM). About 10% of known cases of diabetes in the United States are type 1.

• Type 2 diabetes was previously called non-insulin-dependent diabetes mellitus (NIDDM). About 90% of all known cases of diabetes in the United States are type 2.

• "Other specific types" is the broad term used for classifying patients who have unusual causes of diabetes due to certain diseases of the pancreas, hormonal syndromes, drugs, rare conditions involving the insulin receptor, and other genetic syndromes.

• GDM is diabetes diagnosed during pregnancy. If the diabetes persists after pregnancy, the patient should be reclassified.

■ Distinguishing clinical characteristics of these categories of glucose intolerance are summarized in Table 1.1. A more detailed listing of disorders falling into the "other specific types" category is presented in Table 1.2.

■ Candidates for screening tests for diabetes include:

• all individuals ≥ age 45

• individuals who are obese (≥120% desirable body weight, BMI ≥27 kg/m²)

- adults with first-degree relatives with diabetes
- members of high-risk ethnic groups (Native Americans, Hispanics, Asian Americans, or African Americans)
- women with previous GDM or a history of babies >9 lb at birth
- individuals with hypertension or dyslipidemia (HDL cholesterol ≤35 mg/dl and/or triglycerides ≥250 mg/dl)
- individuals with previously identified IFG or IGT

■ Indications and criteria for screening tests are presented in Table 1.3.

■ A diagnosis of diabetes can be made on the basis of an elevated random plasma glucose concentration plus signs and symptoms of diabetes, an elevated fasting plasma glucose (FPG) concentration, or a properly performed oral glucose tolerance test (OGTT). In contrast to past practice, the FPG is the test of choice because of its simplicity and accuracy. Using the previous diagnostic criteria, some patients would be diagnosed as having diabetes based on an OGTT but would not meet the diagnostic criteria of FPG ≥140 mg/dl. The diagnostic level for diabetes on the FPG has been reduced to ≥126 mg/dl, which brings the FPG and OGTT results into much better concordance.

■ In nonpregnant adults, the diagnosis of diabetes mellitus is based on one of the following tests:

- a random plasma glucose level ≥200 mg/dl (11.1 mmol/l) plus classic symptoms of diabetes mellitus, including polydipsia, polyuria, polyphagia, and weight loss
- a fasting plasma glucose ≥126 mg/dl (7.0 mmol/l)
- a 2-h plasma glucose during an OGTT ≥200 mg/dl (11.1 mmol/l).

■ In the absence of unequivocal hyperglycemia with acute metabolic decompensation, the results should be confirmed by repeat testing on a different day.

■ Some patients do not meet these criteria, but their test results are not completely normal, either. They are classified as follows:

- IFG = FPG ≥110 and <126 mg/dl
- IGT = 2-h OGTT plasma glucose ≥140 and <200 mg/dl

■ The standard OGTT is not necessary for diagnosis of diabetes mellitus and should rarely be done.

■ Normal plasma glucose values for nonpregnant adults are given in Table 1.4. Diagnostic criteria for diabetes mellitus and other categories of glucose intolerance are presented in Table 1.5.

■ It is particularly important to screen pregnant women for the presence of GDM because 60,000–90,000 women with the disease give birth each year, and GDM is associated with increased perinatal morbidity and mortality. Screening for GDM is normally done between the 24th and 28th wk of pregnancy. The small subset of women who are <25 years of age, are of normal body weight, have no first-degree relatives with diabetes, and are Caucasian have a low risk of GDM and need not be screened. This exclusion from screening represents a change from the previous recommendation to screen all pregnant women.

■ The criteria for diagnosis of GDM were proposed by O'Sullivan and Mahan in 1964 and they remain unchanged in the new recommendations. A screening test is done using a 50-g oral glucose load followed by a 1-h plasma glucose measurement. The patient need not be fasting for this test. A value ≥140 mg/dl leads to a follow-up diagnostic test using a 100-g glucose load OGTT over 3 h. Criteria for diagnosis of GDM are summarized in Table 1.6.

■ Before initiating treatment for newly diagnosed diabetes, a complete evaluation should be made to determine:

• type of diabetes
• presence of underlying diseases that need further evaluation
• presence of complications of diabetes

■ Guidelines for evaluations during office visits are given in Table 1.7.

Diagnosis and Classification

Diabetes mellitus is a chronic disorder characterized by abnormalities in the metabolism of carbohydrate, protein, and fat. After some time, it is often accompanied by microvascular, macrovascular, neuropathic, and complications. It is now recognized that diabetes mellitus encompasses a group of genetically and clinically heterogeneous disorders in which glucose intolerance is the common denominator. Thus, although diabetes mellitus affects the metabolism of all body fuels, its diagnosis depends on identification of specific plasma glucose abnormalities.

Because the syndrome of diabetes mellitus encompasses many disorders that differ in pathogenesis, natural history, and responses to treatment, it is important that clinicians and researchers use commonly accepted terminology as well as standardized classification and diagnostic criteria when categorizing patients with glucose intolerance. In July 1997, the American Diabetes Association published new diagnostic and classification criteria replacing the criteria of the National Diabetes Data Group published in 1979. The new criteria were necessary to reflect improved knowledge over the intervening years and to correct common misuse of the previous classification terminology, which was based on treatment rather than pathogenesis.

TYPES OF DIABETES MELLITUS AND OTHER CATEGORIES OF GLUCOSE INTOLERANCE

The classification of diabetes mellitus (Table 1.1) includes four clinical classes: type 1 diabetes, type 2 diabetes, other specific types of diabetes, and gestational diabetes mellitus (GDM). Hyperglycemia not sufficient to meet diagnostic criteria for diabetes is categorized as either impaired fasting glucose (IFG) or impaired glucose tolerance (IGT), depending on whether it is identified on a fasting glucose specimen or after an oral glucose tolerance test (OGTT). The new classification recognizes that a specific type of diabetes may have different stages with varying degrees of hyperglycemia and that the classification should not be determined by the degree or treatment of hyperglycemia. (Fig. 1). The varying stages of hyperglycemia within one type of diabetes mean that at a given point in time it may be difficult to classify an individual patient based on clinical characteristics. Another more minor change is the use of Arabic numerals rather than Roman numerals for type 1 and type 2.

Table 1.1 Types of Diabetes Mellitus and Other Categories of Abnormal Glucose Metabolism

Clinical Classification	Clinical Characteristics
Type 1, immune-mediated	Usually these patients have abrupt onset of polyuria and polydipsia before age 30 and present with ketosis or ketoacidosis. Although they may have a "honeymoon" period at this stage, they are otherwise dependent on insulin treatment for survival. In adulthood the immune destruction of the β-cell may not be severe enough to make insulin treatment essential for survival in the early stages of the disease.
Type 2 diabetes	Usually these patients are over age 30 at diagnosis and are often identified during routine screening without having any symptoms of diabetes. They are not prone to ketoacidosis except with severe physical stress. Their disease is slowly progressive and the treatment necessary to control hyperglycemia varies over time. They may require insulin treatment. Complications of diabetes may be present at diagnosis. These patients are usually obese and have a strong family history of type 2 diabetes.
Other specific types	The presentation in these patients varies greatly depending on the underlying disorder. A careful medication and family history will help identify these patients.
Impaired fasting glucose (IFG)/Impaired glucose tolerance (IGT)	These patients have either fasting or glucose tolerance test results above normal but not diagnostic of diabetes. They should be monitored closely because they have an increased risk of developing diabetes.
Gestational diabetes mellitus (GDM)	Diabetes diagnosed during pregnancy.

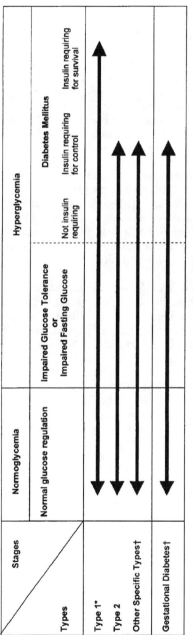
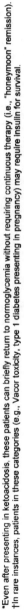

	Stages	Normoglycemia		Hyperglycemia			
					Diabetes Mellitus		
Types		Normal glucose regulation	Impaired Glucose Tolerance or Impaired Fasting Glucose	Not insulin requiring	Insulin requiring for control	Insulin requiring for survival
Type 1*						
Type 2						
Other Specific Types†						
Gestational Diabetes†						

*Even after presenting in ketoacidosis, these patients can briefly return to normoglycemia without requiring continuous therapy (i.e., "honeymoon" remission).
†In rare instances, patients in these categories (e.g., Vacor toxicity, type 1 diabetes presenting in pregnancy) may require insulin for survival.

Figure 1.1 Disorders of glycemia: etiologic types and stages.

TYPE 1 DIABETES

Type 1 diabetes was previously called insulin-dependent diabetes mellitus (IDDM; type I) or juvenile-onset diabetes. There are two subgroups of type 1 diabetes: the more common immune-mediated class and an unusual idiopathic class. Patients with type 1 diabetes mellitus have severe insulinopenia and are prone to the development of ketoacidosis. Most often at diagnosis, type 1 patients are lean, have experienced recent weight loss and symptoms of excessive thirst and urination, and are ketotic or in ketoacidosis. In the stage of complete evolution of the disease, patients with type 1 diabetes mellitus are dependent on exogenous insulin injections to prevent ketoacidosis and death.

Type 1 diabetes is estimated to account for ~10% of all known cases of diabetes mellitus in the U.S. The prevalence is lower among nonwhite than white populations. Although type 1 diabetes may occur at any age, the major peak of onset occurs at about age 11 or 12, and nearly all patients diagnosed before age 20 have this type of diabetes. However, while exact prevalence remains to be established, many Hispanic and African American youths with onset of diabetes before age 20 have type 2 diabetes.

Type 1 immune-mediated diabetes mellitus has strong human leukocyte antigen (HLA) associations, indicating an inherited predisposition to the disease. Early in the disease process, markers of immune destruction of the β-cell are found, including islet cell autoantibodies (ICAs), autoantibodies to insulin (IAAs), and autoantibodies to glutamic acid decarboxylase (GAD_{65}). Beta cell destruction occurs at varying rates, usually more rapidly in younger patients, which accounts for the usual abrupt, classical clinical manifestations; and more slowly in adults, which may lead to the mistaken clinical classification of type 2 diabetes.

Type 1 idiopathic diabetes is a poorly defined class in which the patients are prone to ketoacidosis, but have no evidence of autoimmunity and are most often of African American or Asian ethnic background. The need for insulin therapy may fluctuate in these patients.

TYPE 2 DIABETES

Type 2 diabetes was previously called non-insulin-dependent diabetes mellitus (NIDDM; type II) or adult-onset diabetes. Patients with this class of diabetes treated with insulin were sometimes mistakenly labeled as IDDM in the previous classification terminology. It is hoped that the new classification will avoid this confusion. Patients with type 2 diabetes have residual insulin secretory capacity, although insulin levels are inadequate to overcome the concomitant insulin resistance. As a result, hyperglycemia ensues. Most of these patients are obese and may not have any symptoms of diabetes at the time of diagnosis.

In later stages, insulin secretion diminishes; the patient becomes more hyperglycemic and may have typical diabetic symptoms of excessive thirst and urination. The lack of symptoms often results in a delay in diagnosis, and therefore the patient may have significant diabetic complications present at the time of diagnosis. This problem points out the importance of a diabetes screening program. Type 2 diabetes has a higher prevalence in nonwhite ethnic groups. Characteristics of type 2 diabetes follow.

- Type 2 diabetes can occur at any age, but is usually diagnosed after age 30.
- The age of clinical presentation may be decreasing in some ethnic groups.
- Although about 80% of patients are obese or have a history of obesity at the time of diagnosis, type 2 diabetes can occur in nonobese individuals as well, especially in the elderly.
- Patients with type 2 diabetes may or may not present with classic symptoms of diabetes mellitus (polydipsia, polyuria, polyphagia, and weight loss).
- Patients with type 2 diabetes are not prone to develop ketoacidosis except during periods of severe stress, such as those caused by infections, trauma, or surgery.
- Patients with type 2 diabetes may present with microvascular and macrovascular chronic complications.
- Type 2 diabetes is associated with defects in both insulin secretion and insulin action.

Although patients with type 2 diabetes are not dependent on exogenous insulin injections for survival, many patients require insulin treatment for adequate glycemic control. Insulin may also be needed temporarily for control of stress-induced hyperglycemia.

Type 2 diabetes accounts for about 90% of the diabetic patients in the United States. The prevalence of diagnosed type 2 diabetes mellitus in the United States is about 10.3 million people. There are, most likely, about 5.4 million undiagnosed cases. The prevalence of type 2 diabetes is markedly increased among Native Americans, African Americans, and Hispanics. The prevalence rate increases with age and degree of obesity. There is evidence that the number of new cases diagnosed each year is increasing.

The exact etiology of type 2 diabetes remains unknown. It appears to be a heterogeneous disorder, and both genetic and environmental factors are important. Although type 2 diabetes is not associated with specific HLA tissue types, identical twin studies indicate that there is 50–75% concordance for this disease. The exact genetics appear to be complex and have not been defined. Unlike in type 1 diabetes, circulating ICAs are not present. Intake of excessive calories leading to weight gain and obesity is probably an important factor in the pathogenesis of type 2 diabetes. In fact, obesity, particularly visceral obesity, has been singled out as a most powerful risk factor, and even small weight losses are associated with a change in plasma glucose levels toward normal in many patients with this type of diabetes. A sedentary lifestyle has also been linked to an increased propensity to develop type 2 diabetes. The insulin resistance syndrome, hyperinsulinemia, and IGT are all strong risk factors for developing type 2 diabetes, as is GDM.

OTHER SPECIFIC TYPES OF DIABETES

This category contains the smallest number of patients and may represent <3% of people with diabetes. Table1.2 lists the disorders included in this category. Although this is a small subset of patients with diabetes, correct identification of these patients is important because the treatment is often different. Recognition of the patients in this group requires clinical alertness to identify the examination features or historical differences that lead to the correct diagnosis.

In the previous classification system, there were families in which diabetes was present in children, adolescents, and adults and in which an autosomal dominant inheritance had been established. This form of diabetes was referred to as maturity-onset diabetes of the young (MODY) and was considered a subtype of type 2 diabetes. In the new classification system, MODY is grouped under the heading of other specific types because it is now known that there are several distinct genetic defects of β-cell function responsible for these types of diabetes, and there are minimal or no defects in insulin action that are the hallmark of type 2 diabetes. To date, abnormalities of three different functional genes on different chromosomes have been identified. Each abnormality leads to impaired insulin secretion.

Another change in the classification system is the removal of the class "malnutrition-related diabetes," because there is no convincing evidence that protein deficiency causes diabetes. Many patients previously in this class have fibrocalculous pancreatopathy as the cause of their diabetes. This form of diabetes is common in tropical countries but rare in the United States.

IMPAIRED FASTING GLUCOSE AND
IMPAIRED GLUCOSE TOLERANCE

IFG and IGT are the terms used to describe individuals who have plasma glucose levels that are higher than normal but lower than those considered diagnostic for diabetes mellitus. The importance of this category is that it represents a risk factor for future diabetes and cardiovascular disease. Approximately 25% of these patients eventually develop diabetes mellitus. These patients do not develop the microvascular complications of diabetes unless their hyperglycemia progresses to levels diagnostic of diabetes.

Table 1.2 Other Specific Types of Diabetes Mellitus

- Genetic defects of β-cell function
  - Chromosome 20, HNF-4α (MODY1)
  - Chromosome 7, glucokinaise (MODY2)
  - Chromosome 12, HNF-1α (MODY3)
  - Mitochondrial DNA
  - Mutant insulins
  - Hyperproinsulinemia
  - Others
- Genetic defects in insulin action
  - Type A insulin resistance
  - Leprechaunism
  - Rabson-Mendenhall syndrome
  - Lipoatrophic diabetes
  - Others
- Diseases of the exocrine pancreas
  - Pancreatitis
  - Trauma/pancreatectomy
  - Neoplasia
  - Cystic fibrosis
  - Hemochromatosis
  - Fibrocalculous pancreatopathy
  - Others
- Endocrinopathies
  - Acromegaly
  - Cushing's syndrome
  - Glucagonoma
  - Pheochromocytoma
  - Hyperthyroidism
  - Somatostatinoma
  - Aldosteronoma
  - Others
- Drug- or chemical-induced
  - Vacor
  - Pentadidine
  - Nicotinic acid
  - Glucocorticoids
  - Thyroid hormone
  - Diazoxide
  - β-adrenergic agonists
  - Thiazides
  - Dilantin
  - α-interferon
  - Others
- Infections
  - Congenital rubella
  - Cytomegalovirus
  - Others
- Uncommon forms of immune-mediated diabetes
  - "Stiff-man" syndrome
  - Anti-insulin receptor antibodies
  - Others
- Other genetic syndromes sometimes associated with diabetes
  - Down's syndrome
  - Klinefelter's syndrome
  - Wolfram's syndrome
  - Friedreich's ataxia
  - Huntington's chorea
  - Laurence-Moon-Biedl syndrome
  - Myotonic dystrophy
  - Porphyria
  - Prader-Willi syndrome
  - Others

HNF, hepatocyte nuclear factor.

GESTATIONAL DIABETES MELLITUS

The term GDM is used to describe glucose intolerance that has its onset or is first detected during pregnancy. Women with known diabetes mellitus before conception are not part of this class. Neither are the rare and exceptional cases of typical, classical type 1 diabetes with acute onset any time during pregnancy, and typical, symptomatic type 2 diabetes with onset in the *first* 3 mo of pregnancy. GDM occurs in about 2–4% of pregnant women, usually during the second or third trimester, when levels of insulin-antagonist hormones increase and insulin resistance normally occurs. In normal pregnancy, increased insulin secretion compensates for the insulin resistance.

DIAGNOSIS OF DIABETES MELLITUS AND OTHER CATEGORIES OF GLUCOSE INTOLERANCE

The prevalence of undiagnosed diabetes mellitus in the United States is about 3% of the population, and the currently recommended diagnostic tests for diabetes are neither 100% specific nor 100% sensitive. Based on these facts, it is generally agreed that the risk to the patient of inappropriate diagnosis outweighs the benefits to be gained from screening tests for diabetes in the general community. However, screening high-risk individuals is appropriate.

INDICATIONS FOR SCREENING FOR DIABETES MELLITUS

The recommended screening test for nonpregnant adults is a fasting plasma glucose (FPG) determination. Evaluation for diabetes mellitus should be limited to nonpregnant individuals with a high risk of developing diabetes (Table 1.3).

It is particularly important to screen pregnant women for the presence of GDM because 60,000–90,000 women with the disease give birth each year, and GDM is associated with increased perinatal morbidity. Screening for GDM is normally done between the 24th and 28th wk of pregnancy. The small subset of women who are <25 years of age, are of normal body weight, have no first-degree relatives with diabetes, and are Caucasian have a low risk of GDM and need not be screened. This exclusion from screening represents a change from the previous recommendation to screen all pregnant women.

Table 1.3 Criteria for Testing for Diabetes

- Candidates for screening tests for diabetes include:
  - all individuals ≥ age 45
  - individuals who are obese (≥120% desirable body weight, BMI ≥27 kg/m^2)
  - individuals with first-degree relatives with diabetes
  - members of high-risk ethnic groups (Native Americans, Hispanics, Asian Americans, or African Americans)
  - women with previous GDM or a history of babies >9 lb at birth
  - individuals with hypertension or dyslipidemia (HDL cholesterol ≤35 mg/dl and/or triglycerides ≥250 mg/dl)
  - individuals with previously identified IFG or IGT

Table 1.4 Normal Plasma Glucose Values for Nonpregnant Adults After 75-g Oral Glucose Load

Fasting	<110 mg/dl (<6.0 mmol/l)
30 min	30 min <200 mg/dl (<11.1 mmol/l)
60 min	60 min <200 mg/dl (<11.1 mmol/l)
90 min	90 min <200 mg/dl (<11.1 mmol/l)
120 min	120 min <140 mg/dl (<7.8 mmol/l)

After parturition, patients with GDM should be followed closely. In most cases, glucose tolerance in women with GDM returns to normal after delivery. Within 5–15 years after parturition, however, 40–60% of women with GDM develop type 2 diabetes mellitus.

DIAGNOSTIC CRITERIA FOR DIABETES MELLITUS

A diagnosis of diabetes can be made on the basis of a random plasma glucose concentration plus signs and symptoms of diabetes, a FPG concentration, or a properly performed OGTT. Normal plasma glucose values for nonpregnant adults are given in Table 1.4. Diagnostic criteria for diabetes are presented in Table 1.5.

In contrast to past practice, the FPG is the test of choice because of its simplicity, accuracy, and reproducibility. Using the previous diagnostic criteria, some patients would be diagnosed as having diabetes based on an

Table 1.5 Diagnostic Criteria for Diabetes Mellitus

- Symptoms of diabetes plus casual plasma glucose concentration ≥200 mg/dl (11.1 mmol/l). Casual is defined as any time of day without regard to time since last meal. The classic symptoms of diabetes include polyuria, polydipsia, and unexplained weight loss.

  or
- FPG ≥126 mg/dl (7.0 mmol/l). Fasting is defined as no caloric intake for at least 8 h.

  or
- 2-h plasma glucose ≥200 mg/dl (11.1 mmol/l) during an OGTT. The test should be performed as described by the World Health Organization using a glucose load containing the equivalent of 75 g anhydrous glucose dissolved in water.
- In the absence of unequivocal hyperglycemia with acute metabolic decompensation, these criteria should be confirmed by repeat testing on a different day. The third measure (OGTT) is not recommended for routine clinical use.

OGTT but would not meet the diagnostic criteria of FPG ≥140 mg/dl. The diagnostic level for diabetes on the FPG has been reduced to ≥126 mg/dl, which brings the FPG and OGTT results into much better concordance. The diagnostic levels selected also have been shown in several studies to be very close to the cutoff points at which microvascular complications of diabetes begin to develop, providing some validity for the importance of this degree of hyperglycemia. Although positive urine glucose tests are strongly suggestive of diabetes in symptomatic patients, they should never be used for the definitive diagnosis of diabetes mellitus.

In nonpregnant adults, the diagnosis of diabetes mellitus is based on one of the following tests:

- a random plasma glucose level ≥200 mg/dl (11.1 mmol/l) plus classic symptoms of diabetes mellitus, including polydipsia, polyuria, polyphagia, and weight loss
- a FPG ≥126 mg/dl (7.0 mmol/l)
- a 2-h plasma glucose ≥200 mg/dl (11.1 mmol/l) during an OGTT

In the absence of unequivocal hyperglycemia with acute metabolic decompensation, the results should be confirmed by repeat testing on a different day.

Some patients do not meet these criteria, but their test results are not completely normal, either. They are classified as follows:

- IFG = FPG ≥110 and <126 mg/dl
- IGT = 2-h OGTT plasma glucose ≥140 and <200 mg/dl

ORAL GLUCOSE TOLERANCE TEST

The standard OGTT is not necessary for diagnosis of diabetes mellitus and should rarely be used. The OGTT is useful only if done with strict adherence to proper methods (assurance of a diet adequate in carbohydrate, i.e., 150 g/day for 3 days; absence of underlying illness; and absence of interfering drugs). OGTTs have been used extensively to establish the incidence and prevalence of diabetes in population-based studies. However, OGTTs are of limited value in making the diagnosis of diabetes in a given individual because of the variability from test to test. The OGTT should not be done if FPG >126 mg/dl.

The OGTT is done using a 75-g oral glucose load. Test results at several times are no longer used for diagnosis during the OGTT. Rather, the 2-h plasma glucose value alone is used.

CRITERIA FOR DIAGNOSIS OF GDM

The criteria for diagnosis of GDM were proposed by O'Sullivan and Mahan in 1964 and they remain unchanged in the new recommendations.

Table 1.6 Diagnosis of Gestational Diabetes Mellitus

After a **100-g** oral glucose load, diagnosis of GDM may be made if two plasma glucose values equal or exceed:

Fasting	105 mg/dl	(5.8 mmol/l)
1-h	190 mg/dl	(10.5 mmol/l)
2-h	165 mg/dl	(9.2 mmol/l)
3-h	145 mg/dl	(8.1 mmol/l)

A screening test is done using a 50-g oral glucose load followed by a 1-h plasma glucose measurement. The patient need not be fasting for this test. A value ≥140 mg/dl leads to a follow-up diagnostic test using a 100-g glucose load OGTT over 3 h. Table 1.6 lists the diagnostic criteria. During normal pregnancy, FPG levels tend to decrease, while postglucose load levels tend to increase. Thus, criteria for diagnosis of GDM are adjusted appropriately and are calculated to provide maximum sensitivity (with a corresponding loss of specificity) to diagnose diabetes during pregnancy. Exceeding two or more of the glucose concentrations noted in Table 1.6 has been demonstrated to cause increased risks to the fetus.

EVALUATION AND CLASSIFICATION OF PATIENTS BEFORE TREATMENT

Before therapy is initiated to treat diabetes mellitus, the patient should have a complete medical evaluation and be classified appropriately.

EVALUATION OF THE PATIENT

A complete medical evaluation before initiating therapy helps the physician classify the patient, determine the possible presence of underlying diseases that may require further study, and detect the presence of complications frequently associated with diabetes mellitus (see Chapter 5, Detection and Treatment of Complications). Table 1.7, a reminder list for the medical evaluation, is presented on page 16.

CLASSIFICATION OF THE PATIENT

The patient should not be classified until all data necessary for making the determination are available. Generally, a reasonably good initial assignment of the patient can be made on the basis of a complete personal and family history and diagnostic test results. The most important dis-

Table 1.7 Office Guide to Initial Evaluation

Once diagnosis of diabetes mellitus has occurred, the patient should have a complete evaluation, including a search for the presence of complications frequently associated with diabetes. The following is a reminder list for the complete *initial* evaluation.

Medical History

- Symptoms
- Results of laboratory tests and special examination results related to the diagnosis of diabetes
- Prior glycated hemoglobin records
- Eating patterns, nutritional status, and weight history; growth and development in children and adolescents
- Details of previous treatment programs, including nutrition and diabetes self-management training
- Current treatment of diabetes, including medications, meal plan, and results of glucose monitoring and patients' use of data
- Exercise history
- Frequency, severity, and cause of acute complications such as ketoacidosis and hypoglycemia
- Prior or current infections, particularly skin, foot, dental, and genitourinary
- Symptoms and treatment of chronic complications associated with diabetes
- Other medications that may affect blood glucose levels
- Risk factors for atherosclerosis
- History and treatment of other conditions, including endocrine and eating disorders
- Family history of diabetes and other endocrine disorders
- Gestational history
- Lifestyle, cultural, psychosocial, educational, and economic factors that may influence the management of diabetes

Physical Examination

- Height and weight (and comparison to norms in children and adolescents)
- Sexual maturation (during peripubertal period)
- Blood pressure determination, including orthostatic measurements when indicated, and comparison to age-related norms
- Ophthalmoscopic examination, preferably with dilation
- Oral examination
- Thyroid palpation
- Cardiac examination
- Abdominal examination
- Evaluation of pulses by palpitation and with auscultation
- Hand/finger examination
- Foot examination
- Skin examination
- Neurological examination

Laboratory Evaluation

- FPG (a random plasma glucose level may be obtained in an undiagnosed symptomatic patient for diagnostic purposes)
- Glycated hemoglobin
- Fasting lipid profile, including total cholesterol, HDL cholesterol, triglycerides, and LDL cholesterol
- Serum creatinine
- Urinalysis for glucose, ketones, protein, and evidence of infection
- Determination for microalbuminuria
- Urine culture if evidence of infection is present
- Thyroid function test(s) when indicated

tinguishing characteristics of diabetes mellitus are presented in Table 1.1. Patients should not be classified on the basis of age alone or on whether or not they are taking insulin therapy.

A major problem in classification is that it is sometimes difficult to assign the patient to a particular type of diabetes mellitus (i.e., type 1 or type 2). For example, the normal-weight type 2 patient who has been taking insulin often looks like a type 1 patient. Another example is the newly diagnosed child or adolescent who is a member of a family with an autosomal dominant form of inheritance of diabetes (genetic defect of the β-cell, MODY). This patient should not be classified as having type 1 diabetes on the basis of age alone. There are patients with characteristics of type 2 diabetes who may require insulin therapy for glycemic control but are not dependent on insulin to prevent ketoacidosis or to sustain life. These patients should not be classified as having type 1 diabetes simply on the basis of their insulin regimen. There are patients, particularly in adulthood, who have type 1 immune-mediated diabetes but are at a stage in which they still have β-cell function and clinically behave similarly to type 2 diabetes. It is usually not necessary for clinicians to determine the presence of islet cell or other antibodies or the degree of insulin secretion, but if this problem is suspected, these measurements might be of help. There is some evidence that these patients do better when treated with insulin even though they might temporarily respond to an oral agent. In research studies, the measurement of stimulated plasma C-peptide levels after oral or intravenous stimulus is often used as an index of insulin secretion; however, it has not proved to be a useful classification tool for routine use. A history of ketoacidosis or the detection of moderate to strong urine ketones in the presence of hyperglycemia is the most useful indicator of type 1 diabetes mellitus. Although the classification of some patients may thus be problematic, the goal of therapy remains the achievement of near-normal glycemia.

BIBLIOGRAPHY

American Diabetes Association: Report of the expert committee on the diagnosis and classification of diabetes mellitus. *Diabetes Care* 21 (Suppl. 1):S5–S19, 1998

Harris MI, Hadden WC, Knowler WC, Bennett PH: International criteria for the diagnosis of diabetes and impaired glucose tolerance. *Diabetes Care* 8:562–67, 1985

Keen H: Limitations and problems of diabetes classification from an epidemiological point of view. *Adv Exp Med Biol* 189:31–46, 1985

Little RR, England JD, Wiedmeyer HM, McKenzie EM, Pettitt DJ, Knowler WC, Goldstein DE: Relationship of glycosylated hemoglobin to oral glucose tolerance. *Diabetes* 37:60–64, 1988

Modan M, Halkin H, Karasik A, Lusky A: Effectiveness of glycated hemoglobin, fasting plasma glucose, and a single post load plasma glucose level in population screening for glucose intolerance. *Am J Epidemiol* 119:431–44, 1984

National Diabetes Data Group: Classification and diagnosis of diabetes mellitus and other categories of glucose intolerance. *Diabetes* 28:1039–57, 1979

O'Sullivan JB, Mahan CM: Criteria for the oral glucose tolerance test in pregnancy. *Diabetes* 13:278–85, 1964

Proceedings of the Third International Workshop-Conference on Gestational Diabetes Mellitus. *Diabetes* 40 (Suppl. 2):1–201, 1991

Roseman JM, Go RCP, Perkins LL, Barger BD, Bell DH, Goldenberg RL, DuBard MB, Huddleston JF, Sedlacek CM, Acton RT: Gestational diabetes mellitus among African-American women. *Diabetes Metab Rev* 7:93–104, 1991

Simon D, Coignet H, Thibult N: Comparison of glycated hemoglobin and fasting plasma glucose with two-hour post-load plasma glucose in the detection of diabetes mellitus. *Am J Epidemiol* 122:589–93, 1985

World Health Organization: *Diabetes Mellitus: Report of a WHO Study Group*. Geneva, World Health Org., 1985 (Tech. Rep. Ser. no. 727)

Yudkin JS, Alberti KGMM, McLarty DG, Swai ABM: Impaired glucose tolerance: is it a risk factor for diabetes or a diagnostic ragbag? *Br Med J* 301:397–402, 1990

Pathogenesis

Highlights
Pathogenesis

■ Type 2 diabetes is a heterogeneous disorder characterized by diminished liver, muscle, and adipose tissue sensitivity to insulin (insulin resistance) and impaired β-cell function.

■ In type 2 diabetes:

• basal insulin concentration is normal or increased until late in the course of the disease

• insulin secretion in response to intravenous glucose is reduced, but response to other secretagogues is near normal

• insulin secretion in response to oral glucose may be normal or increased in absolute terms, but in relationship to the response in people without diabetes to the same degree of hyperglycemia, insulin secretion is impaired

• insulin resistance is almost always present and usually precedes development of hyperglycemia

• an initial defect in insulin sensitivity can lead to the emergence of a defect in insulin secretion or, conversely, an impairment in β-cell function can lead to impaired insulin action

• in most patients with type 2 diabetes, at the time of diagnosis both insulin resistance and β-cell functional impairment are present, and it is impossible to determine the initial defect

Pathogenesis

YPE 2 DIABETES is a heterogeneous disorder characterized by diminished liver, muscle, and adipose tissue sensitivity to insulin and impaired β-cell function. There has been debate as to whether insulin resistance (impaired insulin action) or impaired insulin secretion is the initial abnormality in the pathogenesis of type 2 diabetes. However, both insulin secretion and insulin action are impaired in people with type 2 diabetes who have moderately severe hyperglycemia with fasting plasma glucose values >180 to 200 mg/dl (>10 to 11.1 mmol/l). Through the years, evidence has accumulated indicating that defects in insulin action can lead to impaired insulin secretion and that impaired insulin secretion and hyperglycemia can decrease insulin action. Thus, once diabetes is well established, it is difficult to determine in an individual patient whether the primary defect was in the β-cell or the response of tissues to insulin. Nonetheless, certain general statements about the pathogenesis of type 2 diabetes can be made.

INSULIN SECRETION

In people without diabetes there are two phases of insulin release observed after an intravenous glucose injection:

- an early phase that occurs within the first few minutes after injection, representing the release of insulin stored within the β-cell
- a later phase that includes newly synthesized insulin

The relative contribution of these two phases to insulin secretion after oral glucose ingestion is not known.

Early in the course of type 2 diabetes, patients usually have normal or elevated fasting plasma insulin levels. These insulin levels reflect augmented insulin secretion in response to insulin resistance and elevated plasma glucose levels. Later in the course of type 2 diabetes, when fasting plasma glucose in the >250 mg/dl range occurs, β-cell function is severely disturbed and fasting insulin levels are diminished.

GLUCOSE-STIMULATED INSULIN RESPONSE

In patients with impaired fasting glucose or glucose tolerance, the total insulin response after either oral or intravenous glucose is usually increased. As the fasting plasma glucose increases, the early phase of insulin secretion is diminished after food ingestion; however, the later phase may be normal or increased. In people with type 2 diabetes with moderate fasting hyperglycemia (140–180 mg/dl), both phases of insulin secretion are diminished. Because of their insulin resistance, even usual levels of insulin secretion are inadequate to maintain normal glucose tolerance. The presence of insulin resistance demands an increase in insulin secretion to maintain normal glucose levels. In people without diabetes, the presence of insulin resistance from obesity, for example, is compensated for by an increase in insulin secretion. When diabetes develops and progresses to more severe fasting hyperglycemia (>180 mg/dl), the insulin secretory response to both oral and intravenous glucose progressively diminishes. Overall, inadequate insulin secretory response to glucose is one hallmark of type 2 diabetes. The genetic and molecular basis of the impaired insulin secretion is not known.

PHYSIOLOGICAL CONSEQUENCES OF IMPAIRED INSULIN SECRETION

The impairment of insulin secretion has important physiological consequences. When the early phase of insulin secretion is reduced, the portal vein insulin concentration remains low after food ingestion and hepatic glucose production is not suppressed. Continued output of glucose by the liver plus the glucose entering the circulation from the intestinal tract lead to excess hyperglycemia. In addition, because of the reduced insulin secretion, glucose uptake by muscle is reduced, accentuating the hyperglycemia. Early in the progression to diabetes, the reduced initial insulin secretion is followed by late enhanced insulin secretion; eventually, the plasma glucose concentration returns to normal, but only at the expense of hyperglycemia and hyperinsulinemia. As the defect in β-cell insulin secretion progresses, even late insulin secretion diminishes. When this occurs, fasting hyperglycemia and overt diabetes develop.

SUMMARY

Early in the course of type 2 diabetes mellitus, in response to insulin resistance basal insulin concentration is normal or increased, even though maximal β-cell function is impaired. In people with impaired glucose tolerance, the total plasma insulin response to a glucose challenge is usually increased, even though the early insulin response is decreased. In patients with type 2 diabetes and moderate to severe hyperglycemia (>180 mg/dl), all phases of insulin secretion are impaired. With fasting plasma glucose between 120–180 mg/dl, the insulin response to glucose is variable and may be increased, normal, or decreased. It generally is inversely correlated with the degree of fasting hyperglycemia. Overall, insulin responses are inappropriately low compared with those that would be achieved in normal subjects with the same plasma glucose concentrations.

INSULIN RESISTANCE

An impairment in endogenous insulin action was first suggested by the observation that many patients with type 2 diabetes have normal or increased plasma insulin responses after glucose ingestion. Subsequently, numerous investigators demonstrated the presence of insulin resistance in most patients with type 2 diabetes by a variety of techniques. The insulin resistance correlated positively with the elevation in fasting plasma glucose concentration. Insulin resistance is now known to be present early in the development of type 2 diabetes. It is found in some relatives of patients with type 2 diabetes and may identify those at risk of developing diabetes.

MECHANISMS OF INSULIN RESISTANCE AT THE CELLULAR LEVEL

In the most general sense, the action of insulin involves two processes. First, insulin binds to a specific receptor located on the cell surface. Second, the binding of insulin to the receptor activates a series of intracellular events, culminating in enhanced glucose transport and stimulation of a variety of intracellular enzymatic pathways. For the sake of simplicity, all intracellular processes involved in insulin action after it binds to its receptor will be referred to as postbinding events.

Binding Abnormalities

Insulin binding to its specific cell surface receptor is the first stage in the mechanism of insulin action. Reduction in binding leads to impaired insulin action. Abnormal binding has been found with mutations in the insulin gene and the receptor gene that modify the structure of each. Patients with antibodies that competitively bind to the receptor have also been identified. Altogether, these abnormalities are rare and account for <1% of patients with diabetes. Although studies on liver, muscle, and adipose tissue from people with type 2 diabetes have demonstrated reduced binding, the reduction is most likely secondary to the hyperinsulinemia also found in these patients and is unlikely to play a major role in the insulin resistance of type 2 diabetes.

Postbinding Abnormalities

Postbinding abnormalities are primarily responsible for the insulin resistance in patients with type 2 diabetes. The defects include a marked decrease in glucose transport and other intracellular processes involved in glucose metabolism, especially insulin-stimulated glycogen synthesis. Insulin-mediated glucose transport is facilitated by a specific insulin regulated glucose transporter (GLUT4) that is present in muscle and adipocytes. The search for the defects responsible for type 2 diabetes is concentrating on identifying postbinding abnormalities of insulin action.

SITES OF INSULIN RESISTANCE

Numerous studies have demonstrated that insulin resistance exists in both hepatic and peripheral tissues. In muscle impairment of glucose uptake secondary to insulin resistance, insulin resistance is manifested by impaired nonoxidative pathways of glucose utilization, primarily glycogen formation, as well as a slight decrease in glucose oxidation. The decrease in insulin-mediated muscle glucose disposal contributes to the excessive rise in plasma glucose concentration after glucose ingestion in patients with type 2 diabetes. In the liver, insulin resistance leads to failure to suppress hepatic glucose production, even in the face of fasting hyperinsulinemia. Basal rates of hepatic glucose production are increased when the fasting plasma glucose exceeds 140 mg/dl, and the increase correlates with the level of fasting plasma glucose. Patients with type 2 diabetes do not demonstrate normal suppression of hepatic glucose output when insulin is infused intravenously at a low concentration. At high infusion concentrations of insulin, hepatic glucose output can be suppressed, indicating partial ability to overcome the insulin resistance.

SUMMARY

In patients with type 2 diabetes, postbinding abnormalities are primarily responsible for the insulin resistance. When impaired binding is present it may be secondary to obesity and hyperinsulinemia and is unlikely to be the primary cause of the insulin resistance. Nonetheless, it may contribute to impaired insulin sensitivity.

PATHOGENIC SEQUENCES LEADING TO TYPE 2 DIABETES

By the time most patients with type 2 diabetes come to medical attention, fasting hyperglycemia is present and defects in insulin action and secretion are well established. At this stage of our knowledge, it is unknown which defect is primary in the development of the disease. Abnormalities in insulin action can result in β-cell failure, and abnormalities in insulin secretion can lead to the development of insulin resistance. Without impairment of insulin secretion, insulin resistance rarely leads to hyperglycemia. The interrelationship between insulin secretion and insulin action is summarized in Fig. 2.1.

The hypothesis assigning the primary defect to β-cell failure proposes the following. As a first abnormality, the insulin secretory response to glucose is delayed. In addition, the pulsatile pattern of insulin secretion observed in patients without diabetes is either absent or diminished in patients with type 2 diabetes. The defective insulin secretory response leads to inadequate suppression of hepatic glucose production and a decrease in glucose uptake by peripheral tissues during the period immediately after glucose ingestion. The resulting postprandial hyperglycemia is a persistent stimulus to insulin secretion and late hyperinsulinemia, which will eventually return the plasma glucose concentration to normal. At this stage, fasting euglycemia is only maintained by an increased plasma insulin concentration.

The hyperinsulinemia causes downregulation of the number of insulin receptors and leads to postbinding defects. This mechanism could cause the development or worsening of insulin resistance. As β-cell deficiency worsens, the insulin secretory response to glucose becomes more deficient and fasting hyperglycemia occurs. The cause of the progressive

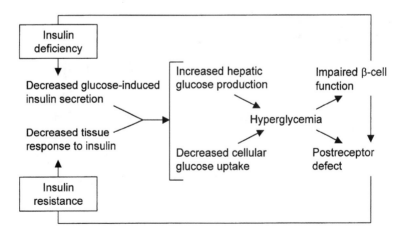

Figure 2.1. Relationship between insulin resistance and insulin secretion in type 2 diabetes mellitus.

nature of the β-cell deficiency is not known, but theoretically could occur for several reasons:

- genetic determinants
- detrimental effects of hyperglycemia on the β-cell
- other metabolic disturbances that occur in diabetes

The hypothesis assigning the primary defect to insulin resistance assumes that insulin resistance is genetically determined and accentuated by obesity. In the basal state, insulin resistance in the liver leads to increased hepatic glucose production, which requires secretion of additional insulin to suppress the liver and prevent fasting hyperglycemia. About 70% of glucose is taken up by insulin-independent tissues, primarily the brain, in the basal state, minimizing the importance of muscle. After glucose ingestion, the insulin-dependent tissues (muscle and liver) become important in the disposal of a glucose load, and hyperglycemia occurs postprandially unless hyperinsulinemia increases glucose disposal. The insulin resistance–induced need for increased insulin secretion in both the fasting and postprandial state eventually cannot be met by the β-cell, and hyperglycemia occurs. The development of hyperglycemia further aggravates both the insulin resistance and β-cell failure (i.e., glucotoxicity).

Either hypothesis is consistent with the typical pattern seen in type 2 diabetes at diagnosis. At that point, both the early and late phases of insulin secretion are impaired, hepatic glucose production is increased in the basal state, and marked muscle insulin resistance is present. Treatment reducing the hyperglycemia may improve both insulin secretion and insulin action, although neither defect returns to normal.

BIBLIOGRAPHY

Haffner SM, Miettinen H: Insulin resistance implications for type II diabetes mellitus and coronary heart disease. *Am J Med* 103:152–62, 1997

Kahn CR: Insulin action, diabetogenes, and the cause of type II diabetes. *Diabetes* 43:1066–84, 1994

Polonsky KS, Sturis J, Bell GI: Non-insulin-dependent diabetes mellitus—a genetically programmed failure of the beta cell to compensate for insulin resistance. *N Engl J Med* 334:777–83, 1996

Reaven GM: Pathophysiology of insulin resistance in human disease. *Physiol Rev* 75:473–86, 1997

Taylor SI, Accili D, Imai Y: Insulin resistance or insulin deficiency: which is the primary cause of NIDDM? *Diabetes* 43:735–40, 1994

Management

Special Therapeutic Problems
    Pregnancy
    Surgery
Assessment of Treatment Efficacy
    Office Methods
    Self-Monitoring

Highlights Management

Therapeutic Objectives and Plan

■ The two major management goals of type 2 diabetes mellitus are to:

- achieve normal metabolic control
- prevent microvascular and macrovascular complications

■ Specific goals of therapy are to:

- eliminate symptoms
- optimize metabolic parameters
- assist the patient to achieve and maintain reasonable body weight
- improve cardiovascular risk factors
- prevent and treat microvascular complications
- achieve optimal overall health and well-being

■ Recommended treatment modalities include:

- dietary modification
- regular physical activity
- pharmacologic intervention with either an oral hypoglycemic agent or insulin

■ Individualize therapy based on patient age, other illnesses, lifestyle, financial restrictions, self-management skills learned, and level of patient motivation.

■ Recommendations for glycemic control are found in Table 3.1.

■ Patient education that enhances self-care behaviors is essential for the successful management of type 2 diabetes mellitus.

Nutrition

■ Medical nutrition therapy is an important element in the therapeutic plan for patients with type 2 diabetes. For some, nutrition and exercise are the only interventions needed to control the metabolic abnormalities associated with type 2 diabetes, including hyperglycemia, hyperlipidemia, and hypertension.

■ When the person with diabetes is overweight, total caloric intake should be decreased to produce a lasting weight loss. Caloric restriction itself is usually successful in lowering plasma glucose levels even before substantial weight loss is achieved. Approaches to weight reduction are outlined on pages 39–41.

■ Patients with type 2 diabetes who are of normal weight should eat sufficient calories to maintain that weight and should distribute carbohydrate intake throughout the day to optimize blood glucose control.

■ Recommendations for nutrient content of the diet, including fat, protein, carbohydrates, sugar and fat substitutes, and micronutrients, are presented on pages 41–46.

■ Patients with diabetes have a greater-than-normal prevalence of hyperlipidemia, atherosclerosis, and hypertension. Nutrition recommendations should consider these conditions, yet be individualized.

■ The use of alcohol is discussed on page 48.

■ Successful implementation of a specific nutrition plan requires:
- patient education and behavior modification
- individualization of the meal plan
- continuous follow-up

Early intervention and follow-up with a dietitian greatly facilitates successful nutrition management.

Exercise

■ Unless contraindicated, appropriate physical activity is strongly recommended to maximize the effects of dietary modification.

■ The potential benefits of increased physical activity include:
- improvement in insulin sensitivity and improvement in glucose tolerance
- promotion of weight loss and maintenance of desirable body weight when combined with restricted caloric intake
- improvement of cardiovascular risk factors
- potential reduction in dosage or need for insulin or oral hypoglycemic agents
- enhancement of work capacity
- enrichment of quality of life and improvement in sense of well-being

■ In some patients requiring hypoglycemic medication, potential hazards are associated with increased physical activity, including hypoglycemia during or after exercise.

■ Exercise should be prescribed with caution if the patient has poorly controlled, labile blood glucose levels or is at increased risk because of microvascular and/or cardiovascular complications.

Pharmacologic Intervention

■ When a patient is unable to achieve normal or near-normal glucose levels with dietary changes and exercise, despite adequate education and effort, pharmacologic treatment should be considered.

■ Pharmacologic intervention is an adjunct to and not a substitute for dietary modification and exercise.

■ The choice between oral hypoglycemic agents and insulin should be made with the particular patient in mind, taking into account the:

• initial level of blood glucose
• level of blood glucose control desired
• total clinical context of the patient's disease

• patient's acceptance of the various therapeutic modalities
• patient's age and weight
• patient's ability for self-care management
• patient's level of diabetes education
• patient's level of motivation
• possible contraindication to medication

■ Oral hypoglycemic agents differ from one another in terms of potency, pharmacokinetics, and metabolism (Tables 3.8 and 3.9).

■ One group of oral hypoglycemic agents (sulfonylureas and repaglinide) augments β-cell insulin secretion.

■ Another group of oral agents enhances the glucose-lowering effects of insulin, each one by a unique mechanism.

■ The patient who is most likely to respond to oral agents has:

• had onset of diabetes after age 40
• had diabetes for <5 yr
• never received insulin or has been well controlled on <40 U/day

■ Oral hypoglycemic agents are contraindicated if the patient:

• has type 1 diabetes

• is pregnant or lactating

• has a stressful concurrent condition with significant hyperglycemia

• is allergic to the drugs

■ Side effects of sulfonylureas and repaglinide are relatively uncommon. The principal adverse reaction is hypoglycemia. Elderly patients are more susceptible to hypoglycemia induced by oral agents, particularly when they skip meals and when hepatic, renal, or cardiovascular function is impaired. In these individuals, sulfonylureas should be used with caution.

■ Metformin, acarbose, and troglitazone are alternative choices for oral therapy of type 2 diabetes. Because they do not increase insulin secretion, they are much less likely to cause hypoglycemia than sulfonylureas or repaglinide. Metformin should not be used with impaired renal function. Troglitazone should not be used with serious cardiac or liver disease.

■ Factors that influence the choice of oral hypoglycemic agent are outlined on pages 63–65. When prescribing an oral agent initially, the lowest effective dose should be used, and the dose should be increased on a schedule suited to that agent until desired glycemic control is achieved or until the maximum effective dose is reached. Some patients maintained on low doses of oral hypoglycemic agents can discontinue the agents and control glucose levels with nutrition and exercise. About 10% of patients each year experience secondary failure to sylfonylureas, which may be due to failure of the patient to follow the prescribed dietary plan, progression of disease, or the occurrence of an underlying stressful disease or condition.

■ Control of blood glucose can often be restored after secondary failure of a single agent by addition of a second one with a different mechanism of action.

■ Insulin therapy can achieve satisfactory blood glucose control in patients with type 2 diabetes. However, insulin resistance—particularly in some patients—may be difficult to overcome and may require large quantities of insulin.

■ The insulin prescription depends on the amount of β-cell function remaining, whether oral agents are continued, and the daily glucose pattern as determined by SMBG. Some patients with mild to moderate fasting hyperglycemia may be adequately controlled with one injection of intermediate-acting insulin before breakfast or at bedtime. Many patients require a multidose regimen consisting of short-acting insulin in combination with either intermediate-acting or long-acting insulin.

■ In select patients who have failed to achieve control on oral agents, an injection of intermediate-acting insulin at night has been used in combination with morning administration of a sulfonylurea, metformin, or troglitazone as a transition to insulin treatment.

■ The main complication of insulin treatment is hypoglycemia, but immediate and delayed allergic reactions at the injection site may occur as well.

■ Several drugs in common use today can cause hyperglycemia or hypoglycemia (Table 3.11). When possible, these drugs should be avoided.

Special Therapeutic Problems: Pregnancy and Surgery

■ Ideally, pregnancy in a patient with diabetes should be planned so that conception occurs when the patient has normal fasting, preprandial, and postprandial plasma glucose levels. Patients should obtain preconception counseling from the health care team. Referral should be considered if the plasma glucose level is >120 mg/dl (6.7 mmol/l) at any time during pregnancy.

■ The major principles governing the management of diabetes during surgery are presented in Table 3.14. The objectives of management before, during, and after surgery are to prevent hypoglycemia and hyperglycemia.

Assessment of Treatment Efficacy

■ The therapeutic response to the treatment of diabetes mellitus is monitored by determining effects on glucose and lipid metabolism. Physicians monitor the responses to treatment with determinations of fasting, preprandial, and postprandial plasma glucose levels (an index of day-to-day control) and with assays for glycated hemoglobin (a reflection of degree of glucose control for the preceding 6–12 wk).

■ Patients can determine the effects of therapy by self-monitoring of blood glucose (SMBG) and measurement of urine ketones, when necessary. They can use a daily journal to record food intake, exercise, doses of insulin or oral hypoglycemic agent, symptoms, and results of self-administered blood tests.

■ Problem solving with SMBG makes it possible for many patients to achieve near-normal glycemia.

Management

THERAPEUTIC OBJECTIVES AND PLAN

There are two major management goals for the patient with type 2 diabetes: to achieve near-normal metabolic control, and to prevent microvascular and macrovascular complications. To achieve the first goal, the physician adjusts elements of the treatment plan to produce normal levels of fasting and postprandial plasma glucose, fasting LDL and HDL cholesterol and triglycerides, and glycated hemoglobin. To prevent or delay the onset of microvascular and neuropathic complications of diabetes, it is important to normalize blood glucose levels. To prevent or delay macrovascular complications, it is also important to normalize lipid levels, lower elevated blood pressure to normal, and help the patient to stop smoking and approach desirable body weight.

There is evidence that long-term glycemic control can prevent or ameliorate the microvascular and neuropathic complications of diabetes. The Diabetes Control and Complications Trial (DCCT) demonstrated definitively the beneficial effects of glycemic control in slowing the progression of retinopathy, nephropathy, and neuropathy in type 1 diabetes. Although no large intervention trial in type 2 diabetes has demonstrated a beneficial impact of intensive treatment regimens on complications, it is reasonable to extrapolate the beneficial effects noted in the DCCT to type 2 diabetes. The accelerated atherosclerosis seen in patients with type 2 diabetes may also be ameliorated with normalization of plasma glucose levels over the long term.

A rational approach to the treatment of patients with type 2 diabetes should include measures that will specifically reverse the underlying pathogenic metabolic disturbances that result in hyperglycemia, i.e., insulin resistance and impaired β-cell function. Various approaches may be used. First, it is critical to educate patients and their families on self-care practices necessary to manage diabetes. National standards exist for diabetes education programs, and these should be followed. In addition, a meal plan and exercise program should be developed. Pharmacologic therapy should be instituted if necessary. An approach should be developed to

Table 3.1 Glycemic Control

Biochemical Index	Normal	Goal	Additional Action Suggested
Fasting/preprandial glucose	<110 (<6.0)	80–120 (<6.6)	<80 or >140 (<4.4 or >7.8)
Bedtime glucose	<120 (<6.7)	100–140 (5.6–7.8)	<100 or >160 (<5.6 or >8.9)
HbA$_{1c}$ (%)	<6	<7	>8

Data are mg/dl (mmol/l). Glycated hemoglobin is referenced to a nondiabetic range of 4–6% (mean 5%, SD 0.5%).

make continuous assessment of metabolic control. Within this scheme, careful attention to psychosocial influences and/or behavior-modification techniques are exceptionally valuable. Finally, the physician must have indices that indicate results of attempts at glycemic control (Table 3.1). Although it is recognized that normal glucose levels usually are not achieved, this remains the goal of optimal therapy. Of course, plasma glucose goals should not be achieved at the expense of recurrent episodes of severe hypoglycemia.

If members of the health care team accept these management goals, follow suggested approaches, use the indices of glycemic management, and strive to correct the vascular risk factors of obesity, dyslipidemia, hypertension, and cigarette smoking they will help their patients with type 2 diabetes improve their lifestyle and prevent or delay vascular complications.

BIBLIOGRAPHY

American Diabetes Association: Standards of medical care for patients with diabetes mellitus (Position Statement). *Diabetes Care* 21 (Suppl. 1):S23–31, 1998

DeFronzo RA, Ferrannini E, Koivisto V: New concepts in the pathogenesis and treatment of non-insulin-dependent diabetes mellitus. *Am J Med* 74:52–81, 1983

Gordon T, Castelli WP, Hjortland MC, Kannel WB, Dawber TR: Diabetes, blood lipids and the role of obesity in CHD risk for women: the Framingham study. *Ann Intern Med* 87:393–97, 1977

NUTRITION

Medical nutrition therapy in diabetes is an interactive, collaborative, continuous process of modifying nutrient intake involving the person with diabetes and his or her health care team. It involves:

- assessment: evaluating an individual's usual food intake, metabolic status, lifestyle, and readiness to make changes
- goal setting: prioritizing what needs to be changed and deciding what the person with diabetes is willing to do
- dietary modification and instruction: teaching the person with diabetes to understand the types and portions of foods to include in a healthy diet, how to read a food label, and the role of carbohydrates in glycemic control so he or she can successfully implement a meal plan that improves metabolic status
- evaluation of successful implementation and follow-up: self-monitoring of blood glucose (SMBG) is necessary to evaluate the effects of diet and exercise on glycemic excursions, and routine glycated protein and serum lipid levels provide feedback on macronutrient intake

Medical nutrition therapy is a very important element in the therapeutic plan for individuals with type 2 diabetes. In fact, for many people with mild to moderate diabetes, an appropriate combination of nutrition and exercise is the only therapeutic intervention needed to effectively control the metabolic abnormalities associated with this disease. The goals of medical nutrition therapy in type 2 diabetes are to:

- maintain near-normal blood glucose levels
- normalize serum lipid levels
- attain and maintain a reasonable body weight
- promote overall health

Because of the heterogeneous nature of type 2 diabetes, there is no single prescription for dietary modification that will achieve these goals in all patients. The meal plan must be individualized. Diversity in insulin secretion capacity and insulin resistance, as well as personal characteristics related to lifestyle, age, body weight, and medication regimen, influence strategies chosen to achieve the nutrition goals. Eating habits, attitude, and learning abilities also influence the ability to achieve nutrition goals. Several obstacles to dietary adherence have been identified and should be considered in the dietary assessment and evaluation plan (Table 3.2).

Guidelines for nutritional intervention in individuals with diabetes have been developed that consider the heterogeneity of diabetes (Table 3.3). The success of a particular dietary intervention is evaluated

Table 3.2 Obstacles to Dietary Adherence for Adults with Diabetes

- Negative emotions: attempt to cope by overeating
- Resisting temptation: social events, special foods, cues, or cravings trigger noncompliance
- Eating out: difficult to control portions and ingredients
- Feeling deprived: regret not being able to eat like people without diabetes
- Temptation to relapse: feeling of wanting to give up or take a vacation
- Planning/priorities: it takes too much time to prepare foods on the meal plan; other things get in the way
- Family/friends: support is not offered and/or positive behaviors not modeled

Adapted from Schlundt D, JADA, 94:874, 1994

via metabolic parameters, e.g., daily SMBG results, glycated hemoglobin, and serum lipids, as well as quality of life and body weight. Failure of one intervention strategy may be corrected by using another.

BODY WEIGHT

Body mass index (BMI) is used as a practical definition of body weight relative to health risk. Body mass index is calculated as weight (kg)/height (m²). The U.S. Dietary Guidelines for Americans has defined a healthy weight as BMI = 19–25. A BMI >27 has been generally accepted as a definition of obesity, while a BMI >30 is thought to be indicative of morbid obesity. Because body weight profoundly influences insulin resistance, insulin requirements, and subsequent blood glucose control, an appropriate daily caloric intake is integral to the nutrition plan in type 2 diabetes. However, caloric intake may not require modification if BMI is normal or an individual is unwilling or unable to restrict intake.

A weight history is valuable to identify if controlling body weight is a problem. A 24-h diet recall or 3-day diet history are helpful in evaluating usual daily caloric intake and eating patterns. This assessment will also identify fat, carbohydrate, and protein intake and meal and snack distribution, as well as micronutrients such as iron, sodium, and calcium.

Normal Weight

Approximately 10–20% of people with type 2 diabetes have a normal BMI and may therefore not need their caloric intake modified. Because individuals of normal weight have found a way to balance caloric

Table 3.3 Nutrition Goals, Principles, and Recommendations

Calories
- Sufficient to attain and/or maintain a reasonable body weight for adults, normal growth and development for children and adolescents, and adequate nutrition during pregnancy and lactation

Protein
- 10–20% of daily calories
- No more than adult RDA (0.8 g per kg body wt per day) with evidence of nephropathy

Fat
- Saturated fat <10% of daily calories, <7% with elevated LDL cholesterol
- Polyunsaturated fat up to 10% of total calories
- Remaining total fat varies with treatment goals
- ~30%—normal weight and lipids
- <30%—obese, elevated LDL cholesterol
- ≤40%—elevated triglycerides unresponsive to fat restriction and weight loss
- Predominately monounsaturated fat

Cholesterol
- <300 mg/day

Carbohydrate
- Difference after protein and fat goals have been met
- Percentage varies with treatment goals

Sweeteners
- Sucrose need not be restricted, must be substituted as carbohydrate
- Nutritive sweeteners have no advantage over sucrose and must be substituted as carbohydrate
- Nonnutritive sweeteners approved by the FDA are safe to consume

Fiber
- 20–35 g/day

Sodium
- <3,000 mg/day
- <2,400 mg/day in mild to moderate hypertension

Alcohol
- Moderate usage, i.e., <2 alcoholic beverages daily

Vitamins and Minerals
- Same as the general population

Goals must always be individualized. RDA, recommended dietary allowance.

intake with expenditure, the focus of the nutrition plan can be on modifying other components, such as macro- and micronutrients. Carbohydrate content of the diet and the distribution of carbohydrates between meals and snacks becomes the primary intervention. Carbohydrates have the greatest impact on postprandial blood glucose response. Setting a carbohydrate goal for meals and snacks is one of the best ways to maximize dietary effectiveness. Patients can be taught to increase or decrease carbohydrate intake per meal and/or snack to yield optimal blood glucose results. If they use short-acting insulin they may be able to adjust insulin dose to altered carbohydrate intake. Protein intake need not be modified if it falls within USDA guidelines. Fat intake and proportion of calories from fat should be dictated by the level of dyslipidemia, as well as the level of carbohydrate that optimizes blood glucose.

Occasionally, particularly in the elderly or those individuals with additional medical problems that increase metabolic needs (wound healing, neuropathy, or gastrointestinal disturbances), it may be necessary to increase caloric intake. Care should be taken to provide enough calories, protein, vitamins, and minerals to promote healing and anabolic processes.

Overweight

Approximately 80–90% of people with type 2 diabetes are obese; thus, weight loss is initially the primary treatment goal. Calorie restriction itself may be responsible for improved glucose tolerance, because the loss of as little as 5–10% of body weight improves insulin sensitivity and glucose uptake, reduces insulin secretion, and decreases hepatic glucose production. Weight loss may be most beneficial early in the diagnosis of type 2 diabetes when insulin secretion is greatest. Furthermore, both weight reduction and physical activity improve insulin resistance and may play a role in preventing type 2 diabetes.

Weight reduction can be accomplished by a combination of modest caloric restriction, physical activity, behavior modification of eating habits, and psychosocial support. Although most clinicians agree on this, many seriously overweight individuals find weight loss and, more importantly, weight maintenance, difficult. Genetic predisposition to obesity and possible impaired metabolic and appetite regulation may influence a person's ability to lose weight via any regimen. Furthermore, most individuals will regain lost weight. It has been suggested that such fluctuations in weight are unhealthy for modestly overweight individuals, but little scientific evidence substantiates this concern. On the other hand, the effects of weight gain of as little as 10 kg after age 18 on chronic disease and health are becoming increasingly evident.

Generally, body fatness increases with age, although debate exists over whether this is an effect of aging or decreased muscle mass from lack of exercise. Body fat distributed above the waist increases the risk of developing diabetes, cardiovascular disease, and hypertension. A waist-to-hip ratio >1.0 or waist ≥40 in (102 cm) in men and waist-to-hip ratio >0.8 or waist ≥35 in (88 cm) in women increases risk for cardiovascular mortality.

Because of the psychological and physiological impact of "dieting," obese individuals should be encouraged to attain a reasonable body weight as determined by BMI. Note that reasonable weight or BMI is defined as the weight an individual and health care provider acknowledge as achievable and maintainable, in both the short and long term. This may not be the same as defined desirable or ideal BMI (i.e., <25).

A healthy weight-loss goal is ~2 BMI units or approximately 8–16 lb initially. The U.S. Dietary Guidelines for Americans endorse small weight losses of 1/2 to 1 lb/wk. Not only does an overall weight loss of 5–10 lb improve glucose tolerance, it also reduces blood pressure and serum lipid levels.

A 3,500-kcal deficit will produce a loss of 1 lb of body fat. Daily calorie intake should be evaluated with a diet history and adjusted to produce a modest deficit. Generally, a decrease of 500 calories/day is needed to produce a 1-lb loss of fat/wk. This can vary, however, based on the individual and his or her willingness to restrict intake and/or increase activity. Regular exercise enhances weight loss in dieting individuals and is identified as a predictor for successful weight maintenance.

Because a restriction of <1,200 calories for women and <1,500 calories for men is difficult to adhere to and can be nutritionally inadequate, most individuals will be more successful if they reduce usual daily intake by 250 calories and increase daily activity by 250 calories. If the diet history is unreliable, approximate daily calorie intake can be estimated by multiplying actual weight in lb by a factor of 10–15 (the factor decreases with age and decreasing physical activity level).

Since weight gain in an overweight individual is medically detrimental, and losing weight and keeping it off is extremely difficult, preventing weight gain should be given the same importance as weight loss in an obese individual. A healthy diet plan of moderation combined with daily physical activity is the primary intervention in type 2 diabetes.

Alternative approaches for calorie restriction are possible with individuals who are seriously overweight. Very restrictive low-calorie diets (600–800 kcal/day) are sometimes used in type 2 diabetes. This medically supervised approach generally involves a liquid formula, but may be accomplished with high-quality lean protein sources (1.5 g per kg body wt per day) with vitamin and mineral supplementation. Weight loss is rapid (3–5 lb/wk), and hyperglycemia generally improves within 24 h of implementation. Near-maximum blood glucose improvement is achieved within 10 days of initiating this regimen. However, this approach should be restricted to individuals who are at least 30% above desirable weight (BMI >30). For some, using this regimen for as short a period as 2–12 wk can provide the psychological motivation needed to encourage dietary adherence and may, in fact, improve blood glucose control enough to minimize the need for pharmacological therapy. Alternating a very-low-calorie dietary regimen with a modest caloric reduction has been used successfully in some studies, as has a weekly "day of fasting," and may be a potential alternative for some individuals.

Pharmacotherapy for the treatment of obesity is considered safe and effective in high-risk obese individuals, including those with type 2 diabetes. Each medication has its benefits and risks and needs to be used under close medical supervision. Most people will regain the lost weight once the medication is stopped. Therefore, research into the potential long-term use of these drugs is ongoing. Surgical interventions have been successful in people with a BMI >40. Like pharmacotherapy, surgery is only an adjunct to diet and exercise.

People with type 2 diabetes who take oral hypoglycemic agents or insulin may require a decrease or discontinuation of the medication as calorie restriction is implemented and as weight loss progresses. This may be a gradual reduction with a modestly hypocaloric diet or a rapid reduction (50%) with a very-low-calorie diet. Failure to decrease the dose of medication can compromise weight-loss efforts because hypoglycemia and its treatment increase calorie intake. In addition, some research and considerable anecdotal evidence suggest that excessive doses during insulin therapy may also lead to hunger and overeating, which is counterproductive in obesity.

The results of SMBG provide the necessary feedback to make adjustments in nutrition and medication therapy. Frequent follow-up with a dietitian provides problem-solving techniques and encouragement and supports the weight-loss efforts. This can be done individually or in groups. Appropriate referrals to local hospital programs or other weight-loss programs with qualified staff are useful.

PROTEIN

The recommendation for protein intake in type 2 diabetes is the U.S. recommended dietary allowance (RDA) of 0.8 g per kg body wt per day for adults. Typically, larger amounts are consumed in Western diets (1.2–2.0 g per kg body wt per day). Thus, protein accounts for ~12–20% or more of total calorie consumption. Because excessive protein consumption may aggravate renal insufficiency, 0.8–1.0 g per kg body wt per day may represent an optimal goal in type 2 diabetes. This goal is reflected in the USDA Food Guide Pyramid recommendation of 5–7 oz of lean protein daily. Accomplishing this goal gradually over several months or even years may be necessary since it represents a major alteration in attitude toward protein in the diet. Meat, fish, and poultry are limited to 3–5 oz/day on a 0.8 g/kg regimen. More severe restriction (0.6 g per kg body wt per day) has been suggested to reduce proteinuria and slow the progression of renal failure in patients who exhibit some renal insufficiency. Compliance with such a regimen is difficult, and studies have suggested muscle wasting and loss of totalbody protein can result. Therefore, individuals with diabetes should not consume <0.8 g per kg body wt per day of protein. Increasing evidence suggests that not all proteins have the same effect on the kidneys. Vegetable protein has been shown to result in a lower glomerular filtration rate and renal plasma flow—suggestive of less stress on the kidney than certain animal proteins (i.e., beef). There is limited evidence demonstrating that individuals with type 2 diabetes with lack of insulin secretion to glucose stimuli continue to secrete insulin in response to protein ingestion (specifically, certain amino acids). The glycemic effect of adding or subtracting protein from a given meal or snack can be evaluated with SMBG.

FAT

With protein accounting for 10–20% of total calories, remaining calories will be derived from a combination of fat and carbohydrate. The proportion derived from either depends on the desired medical outcome for each individual patient. Lipid abnormalities common in type 2 diabetes are influenced by carbohydrate and fat content of the diet as well as by body weight, genetics, physical activity, and glycemic control. Hypertriglyceridemia and low HDL cholesterol are the most common lipid abnormalities in type 2 diabetes. This dyslipidemia has been shown to be a significant risk factor for cardiovascular disease in people with and without diabetes.

High-carbohydrate low-fat diets, while recommended by many health organizations and nutrition experts to reduce total and LDL cholesterol, have been shown to increase postprandial blood glucose and triglyceride levels, elevate fasting triglyceride levels, and decrease HDL levels in insulin-resistant type 2 diabetes. The elevated triglyceride levels appear to be secondary to higher circulating insulin concentrations stimulated by high carbohydrate intake. This attribute has sparked concern over the wisdom of recommending a low-fat diet in insulin-resistant type 2 diabetes. Several investigators have shown improved lipid levels and blood glucose control in both short- and long-term studies in which total fat intake approaches 45% of calories and carbohydrate intake is as low as 40% of calories.

Because saturated fat intake should comprise fewer than 10% of total calories and polyunsaturated fats up to 10%, any increase in fat calories should come from monounsaturated fats. Indeed, studies comparing low-fat with low-carbohydrate diets in type 2 diabetes have used monounsaturated fat in amounts up to 25% of calories. Major sources of monounsaturated fat include olive, canola, and peanut oils. However, animal fat, such as that found in beef, pork, and poultry, is nearly one-third monounsaturated fat. Increasing the monounsaturated fat content of the diet without increasing calories can be a challenge that generally requires the professional assistance of a dietitian. Substituting olive and canola oils for other vegetable oils and margarines is primary, but limited, and can be augmented by adding nuts, olives, and avocado to meals and snacks.

Concern that increasing fat intake could potentially lead to weight gain has proved unfounded, as a review of controlled clinical studies using high–monounsaturated fat low-carbohydrate diets demonstrates. Nonetheless, epidemiological studies have documented an increasing incidence of obesity as dietary fat increases. Dietary fat contains more than twice as many calories as either carbohydrate or protein and is thought to be more easily converted into body fat. Since over 80% of people with type 2 diabetes are obese and weight loss and/or maintenance is a primary treatment goal, dietary fat restriction seems a logical first line of dietary therapy in type 2 diabetes. Reducing fat intake in obese individuals will not necessarily lead to reduced calories and weight loss if the individual compensates with low-fat carbohydrate-rich food choices. A low-fat diet without weight loss may or may not result in improved lipid levels in an obese person with type 2 diabetes.

Obese people with diabetes should be given a substantial time period on a reduced fat and calorie plan. If metabolic parameters such as serum lipids and blood glucose control do not improve, then the practitioner should consider a moderate fat increase using monounsaturated fats with a subsequent reduction in carbohydrate intake. Close follow-up and monitoring of metabolic parameters should guide further dietary adjustments.

Saturated fats should make up fewer than 10% of total calories because of their dramatic effect on serum total and LDL cholesterol levels. Currently, adults in the United States consume about 13% of total calories from saturated fat. Saturated fatty acids have been shown to be twice as potent in raising plasma cholesterol as polyunsaturated fats are in lowering them. Saturated fatty acids are predominately found in animal products, but the amount varies between species (Table 3.4). Coconut and palm oils are highly saturated vegetable oils used in baked products, such as cookies and crackers. Whole-milk dairy products and baked goods contribute more to the saturated fat content of the U.S. diet than do meat and meat products. Thus, the most effective way to reduce saturated fat content of the diet is to substitute low-fat milk products, limit meat to lean cuts and reasonable portions, and use baked products made with vegetable oils that have not been hydrogenated.

Cholesterol intake should be limited to <300 mg/day. All animal products, including meat, poultry, eggs, cheese, full-fat dairy products,

Table 3.4 Fatty Acid Composition of Selected Fats (Percentage of Total Lipid)

Type of Fat	MUFA	PUFA	SFA
Vegetable			
Canola (rapeseed)	66	24	5
Coconut	6	2	87
Corn	25	59	13
Olive	74	8	14
Palm	37	9	49
Peanut	46	32	17
Safflower	12	75	9
Soybean	23	58	14
Animal			
Beef	43	4	40
Butter	29	4	62
Chicken	39	22	28
Lamb	42	7	42
Pork	46	11	36
Salmon	35	29	19
Turkey	32	27	29

Data do not total 100%. Additional components include cholesterol and phytosterols. MUFA, monounsaturated fatty acid; PUFA, polyunsaturated fatty acid, SFA, saturated fatty acid.

Adapted from Agriculture Handbook, No. 8 Series, U.S. Department of Agriculture, Human Information service.

and shellfish, contain cholesterol. Consuming low-fat dairy products and lean cuts of meat and limiting eggs to ~4/wk are the most substantial ways to reduce dietary cholesterol intake. It should be noted that while decreasing cholesterol intake reduces serum cholesterol levels, quantitatively, its effect is less than that of lowering saturated fat. The beneficial effect of substituting poultry and fish for red meat is primarily due to the reduced saturated fat content of poultry and fish, since the cholesterol content may be similar. The level of serum cholesterol reduction one can expect from dietary reduction of fat and cholesterol will vary with the individual.

Polyunsaturated vegetable fats are liquid at room temperature but can be hydrogenated to yield a more solid product, such as margarine or shortening. In the process, *trans* fatty acids, which have proven to be as atherogenic as saturated fats in controlled clinical trials, are created. Epidemiological studies have also found an association between the *trans* fatty acid content of the diet and an increased risk of cardiovascular disease. Vegetable oils and soft margarines are preferred polyunsaturated fat sources.

Fish oil contains polyunsaturated fatty acids in the form of omega-3 fatty acids. Omega-3 fatty acids have been proven to have a beneficial effect on cardiovascular disease risk by reducing serum triglycerides and decreasing platelet aggregation. Since both abnormalities are present in type 2 diabetes, it seems logical that fish oil consumption could be beneficial. To date, studies with fish oil capsule supplementation have not shown good results, as blood glucose control worsens. Consuming 8 oz of fish each week has been suggested as a safe and effective alternative. All fish contains some fish oil; however, salmon, albacore tuna, mackerel, and herring are the best sources.

CARBOHYDRATE

The amount and type of carbohydrate that should be included in the diet of a person with type 2 diabetes should be individualized and, as with fat and protein, be driven by the predominant metabolic abnormality one seeks to improve. If LDL and total cholesterol are elevated, then the initial diet plan should restrict fat to 30% or less. This would result in ~50–60% of calories being derived from carbohydrate. The clinician should then carefully evaluate daily blood glucose levels and HbA$_{1c}$ values along with their impact on serum triglycerides and cholesterol to determine if this plan is achieving the desired medical outcomes. If not, a gradual decrease in carbohydrate may be warranted with a subsequent increase in fat, predominantly monounsaturated fat. The USDA Food Guide Pyramid is a good source for recommending carbohydrate choices for individuals with type 2 diabetes. Its emphasis on whole grains, fruits, and vegetables supplies necessary fiber, vitamins, minerals, and antioxidants to the meal plan.

Clinical research investigating the impact of carbohydrate-containing foods on blood glucose response has shown that some differences among carbohydrates do exist. Traditionally, starches and grains were thought to produce a lower glycemic response than sugar-containing foods, such as fruits and sweets. Research has not demonstrated this to be true. The longer chains of glucose molecules present in complex carbohydrates, such as starches, do not necessarily yield a flatter blood glucose response curve than the simple carbohydrates found in sugars. When equal amounts of carbohydrate are compared, no significant difference in glycemic response is seen. Factors such as processing, preparation, and rate of digestion affect the glycemic response of a specific food.

Clinically, the most important determinant of glycemic response to a meal is the total carbohydrate content. Fat and protein contribute little to blood glucose response other than slowing the rate of digestion and absorption of carbohydrate and shifting the response curve to the right. As a result, once the total amount of carbohydrate to be included in the diet is determined, carbohydrate should be distributed between meals and snacks in a pattern than yields the optimal blood glucose responses. Blood glucose testing is crucial in evaluating carbohydrate distribution. Once the optimal distribution is defined, the therapeutic focus shifts to promoting consistent carbohydrate intake in meals and snacks on a daily basis. Patients requiring insulin can adjust short-acting insulin doses to changing carbohydrate consumption.

Fiber is a nondigestible form of carbohydrate that contributes bulk to the diet and appears to slow down the digestion and absorption of carbohydrate. Soluble fiber, such as that found in oat bran and legumes, can blunt postprandial blood glucose responses and reduce serum cholesterol levels. Nonsoluble fiber from wheat bran and many fruits and vegetables has little impact on reducing blood glucose or serum cholesterol, but it is necessary for optimal gastrointestinal function. People with diabetes should consume a daily amount of fiber that meets or exceeds the USDA recommendation of 25 g/day.

Sugar restriction is no longer the primary focus of diet therapy in diabetes. Clinical research has not found sugar-containing foods to be detrimental to blood glucose control when substituted gram for gram for other carbohydrates in the diets of people with diabetes. A modest intake of sugar-containing foods is allowable in the context of a healthy diet. Once again, the USDA Food Guide Pyramid can serve as an excellent guide. Individuals with diabetes can be instructed how to substitute sugary foods using carbohydrate-counting plans or the exchange system. Obese individuals need to be cautioned that high-sugar foods, such as cookies, pastries, and ice creams, are also high in fat and calories. Portion control and understanding how to read food labels is crucial to success.

SUGAR AND FAT SUBSTITUTES

Sorbitol, mannitol, and fructose are commonly used sweeteners that have a lower glycemic effect than either glucose or sucrose (table sugar). Fructose contains the same amount of calories as glucose and sucrose (4 kcal/g); thus, it cannot be used ad libitum, particularly in the hypocaloric diet. The sugar alcohols sorbitol and mannitol have only 2–3 kcal/g, but they are often found in products when extra fat has been added. They may cause gastrointestinal distress, such as bloating and diarrhea, when more than 30 g/day are consumed (10–15 hard candies). Foods containing these sugars must be accounted for in the meal plan.

Noncaloric sweeteners such as aspartame, saccharin, and acesulfame K are more than 200 times sweeter than sugar. They are used in such small quantities that they contribute virtually no calories or nutrition to foods. Their use as tabletop sweeteners and in soft drinks is beneficial in diabetes because they contribute no calories or carbohydrates. However, they may be used in foods that contain other sources of carbohydrates and calories, such as ice cream, cookies, and puddings. These foods need to be worked into the meal plan appropriately.

Fat substitutes currently on the market are derived primarily from carbohydrate or protein. This reduces their caloric value from 9 to 4 kcal/g. However, the use of fat substitutes in yogurt, ice cream, salad dressings, and so on increases the carbohydrate content of the products above their usual level. Individuals should be advised to consider the carbohydrate level when using such foods.

Newer fat substitutes, such as Olestra, are fat replacers made from fat that has been modified to be totally nondigestible and therefore not absorbed. As a result, Olestra adds no fat or fat calories to products. Sugar- and fat-modified foods may be beneficial to people with diabetes by assisting them to reduce their fat, carbohydrate, and calorie intake. However, they are not necessary to follow a healthy diet and should only be suggested as alternatives.

VITAMINS AND MINERALS

There is currently no evidence for an increased need for vitamins or minerals in diabetes above the current RDA. However, antioxidants, such as β-carotene, vitamin E, and vitamin C, have been implicated as potentially valuable in reducing cardiovascular disease risk and cataracts in the general population—both of which are prevalent in type 2 diabetes. Unfortunately, there have been no long-term controlled clinical studies published to date, particularly in people with diabetes, that have shown benefit from antioxidant consumption. It is impossible to obtain the levels of vitamin E that studies show to be potentially beneficial (>100 IU/day) through food intake. Supplementation of vitamin E is considered safe at a level as high as 400 IU/day. However, little benefit is demonstrated above 200 IU/day.

Chromium and its role in preventing and treating type 2 diabetes is still controversial. Chromium potentiates insulin action, and a deficiency of chromium has been implicated in causing insulin resistance characterized by elevated blood glucose levels, triglycerides, and reduced HDL. Supplementation studies with 1,000 µg/day have yielded improved blood glucose control in people with type 2 diabetes. Studies on people without diabetes have shown that supplementation of 200 µg/day may reduce total cholesterol and increase HDL cholesterol. It is possible that chromium supplementation may be of value in chromium-deficient individuals; however, at present there is no good way to evaluate deficiency. Moreover, the long-term effects of chromium supplementation are unknown. Whole-grain products, nuts and seeds, and protein-rich foods are our best sources of chromium, but these can realistically provide only about 50 μg/day.

Sodium recommendations for people with diabetes are no more restrictive than for the general population. Some health authorities recommend no more than 3,000 mg/day of sodium for the general population, while other authorities recommend no more than 2,400 mg/day. For people with mild to moderate hypertension, ≤2,400 mg/day of sodium is recommended. Severe sodium restriction seems to be less valuable than weight loss in controlling hypertension in obese people with type 2 diabetes.

ALCOHOL

Strict abstinence from alcohol is not necessary for patients with diabetes mellitus. In most cases, moderate amounts of alcohol, as recommended for the general population, are allowable in diabetes. Recent studies in the general population have shown reduced cardiovascular disease mortality with moderate alcohol consumption (1–2 drinks/day). This benefit is greatest in people with the highest risk of cardiovascular mortality. Since people with diabetes are at greater risk, there appears little reason to deprive them of the potential benefits of moderate alcohol consumption, which include reduced insulin resistance, increased HDL cholesterol levels, decreased platelet aggregation, and increased fibrinolytic activity. Obviously, alcohol consumption is not recommended for people with conditions such as pregnancy, alcoholism, cirrhosis of the liver, and symptomatic neuropathy.

When alcohol is part of the calorie-controlled meal plan, it is convenient to account for the calories by reducing the patient's fat intake. Before a patient may include alcohol in his or her eating plan, the potential problems associated with alcohol consumption should be considered; e.g., alcohol consumption by a person who is fasting (>5 h) or undernourished may lead to hypoglycemia. This can be a serious problem in patients taking insulin or an oral hypoglycemic agent who skip meals. A patient's ability to follow the prescribed management plan will be impaired if he or she is intoxicated. Additionally, alcohol ingestion may be associated with significant elevations in fasting and postprandial plasma triglyceride levels in people with hypertriglyceridemia.

BIBLIOGRAPHY

American Diabetes Association: Nutrition recommendations and principles for people with diabetes mellitus (Position Statement). *Diabetes Care* 21 (Suppl. 1):S32–35, 1998

American Diabetes Association: Food labeling (Position Statement). *Diabetes Care* 21 (Suppl. 1):S62–63, 1998

American Diabetes Association: Role of fat replacers in diabetes medical nutrition therapy (Position Statement). *Diabetes Care* 21 (Suppl. 1):S64–65, 1998

American Diabetes Association: Translation of the diabetes nutrition recommendations for health care institutions (Position Statement). *Diabetes Care* 21 (Suppl. 1):S66–68, 1998

American Diabetes Association: Detection and management of dyslipidemia in adults with diabetes (Position Statement). *Diabetes Care* 16 (Suppl. 2):106–12, 1993

Bell DSH: Alcohol and the NIDDM patient. *Diabetes Care* 19:509–13, 1996

DCCT Research Group: Expanded role of the dietitian in the Diabetes Control and Complications Trial: implications for clinical practice. *J Am Diet Assoc* 93:758–64, 767, 1993

Franz MJ, Horton ES, Bantle JP, Beebe CA, Brunzell JD, Coulston AM, Henry RR, Hoogwerf BJ, Stacpoole PW: Nutrition principles for the management of diabetes and related complications. *Diabetes Care* 17:490–518, 1994

Mooridian AD, Failla M, Hoogwerf B, Maryniuk M, Wylie-Rosett J: Selected vitamins and minerals in diabetes. *Diabetes Care* 17:464–79, 1994

U.S. Department of Agriculture: *The Food Guide Pyramid*. Hyattsville, MD, Human Nutrition Information Service, 1992

EXERCISE

Exercise in type 2 diabetes can be a useful therapeutic tool. To be effective, an exercise regimen requires individualization and monitoring. Specific precautions need to be taken in some individuals to ensure benefit and minimize risk.

Both obesity and inactivity contribute to the development of glucose intolerance in the person genetically predisposed to diabetes. Regular exercise may delay or prevent type 2 diabetes onset in high-risk populations.

POTENTIAL BENEFITS OF EXERCISE

Regular exercise in type 2 diabetes has the potential to:

- reduce cardiovascular risk factors such as hyperlipidemia and hypertension
- augment weight-reduction diets
- improve blood glucose control by enhancing insulin sensitivity
- reduce dosage or need for insulin or oral medications
- enhance quality of life
- improve psychological well-being

Improved Insulin Sensitivity/Glucose Tolerance

Insulin resistance is a feature of type 2 diabetes mellitus. Exercise enhances insulin sensitivity and increases skeletal muscle glucose uptake, both during and for 48 h after the activity. Thus, repeated bouts of exercise at regular intervals are most beneficial to reduce the glucose intolerance associated with type 2 diabetes. This exercise-induced enhanced sensitivity to insulin occurs without changes in body weight. Unless contraindicated by other health problems, exercise should be a component of the treatment regimen in all people with type 2 diabetes, regardless of whether there is a need for weight reduction.

Exercise may result in a decrease in the amount of insulin or oral agent usually taken. Therefore, careful SMBG is required to minimize hypoglycemia.

Exercise and Weight Reduction

Physical activity is recognized as an important part of weight-reduction programs. In fact, exercise has been identified consistently as the strongest predictor for long-term maintenance of lost weight. Exercise increases energy expenditure to create a greater caloric deficit than a hypocaloric diet alone. Exercise also increases lean body mass (muscle tissue), which helps to maintain the metabolic rate that otherwise declines with loss of body weight. Of particular importance is the fact that aerobic exercise decreases abdominal (central) adiposity. Because central obesity increases cardiovascular risk, this can be of value to patients with type 2 diabetes.

Cardiovascular Conditioning

The value of physical training in ameliorating risk factors for cardiovascular disease has been amply demonstrated in nondiabetic individuals. Exercise is associated with a reduction in circulating levels of VLDL and LDL cholesterol and triglycerides, and increases in levels of HDL cholesterol. Furthermore, exercise is associated with decreases in blood pressure and heart rate both at rest and during exercise, as well as increases in maximum oxygen uptake and total working capacity.

The beneficial effects of exercise on risk factors in patients with type 2 diabetes have not been studied extensively, but it is reasonable to assume that exercise may help to prevent or slow cardiovascular complications in this particularly susceptible group of individuals. Again, however, the cardiovascular and metabolic benefits of exercise are sustained only as the result of the sum of effects of individual bouts of exercise or as a result of long-term changes in body composition.

Psychological Benefits

Exercise training and fitness are often associated with decreased anxiety, improved mood and self-esteem, and an increased sense of well-being. Enhanced quality of life may be a secondary benefit to strength training (increased muscle mass, flexibility, and range of motion), particularly in the aging population in which type 2 diabetes predominates. Regular exercise may improve glucose control in part by providing a coping mechanism for stress.

PRECAUTIONS AND CONSIDERATIONS

Exercise of any kind is safe for most people with type 2 diabetes. However, special precautions should be taken. Because many individuals with type 2 diabetes have led sedentary lives for years, they are frequently deconditioned. Individuals over 35 yr of age not engaged in regular exercise should have a physical examination (including a cardiac stress test) before beginning a vigorous exercise program.

The medical evaluation should include the following:

- determination of glycemic control
- cardiovascular examination (blood pressure, peripheral pulses, bruits, blood lipids, ECG at rest and during exercise if the patient is >35 yr or has a history of cardiovascular disease)
- determination of working capacity (graduated exercise test with measurement of pulse rate response or oxygen consumption)
- neurologic examination
- ophthalmoscopic examination, especially if proliferative retinopathy is present or suspected

Since most people with type 2 diabetes have had the disease for several years before diagnosis, newly diagnosed patients should be examined for hypertension, neuropathy, retinopathy, and nephropathy (Table 3.5). Silent ischemic heart disease can be present without chest pain. Autonomic neuropathy and β-blockers may interfere with maximal heart rate and exercise performance. This is in addition to the already observed 15–20% lower age-matched maximal heart rate found in people with type 2 diabetes. Lower target heart rates and less stressful exercise regimens are recommended in these individuals. Strenuous exercise is contraindicated for patients with poor metabolic control and for those with significant diabetic complications (particularly active proliferative retinopathy, significant cardiovascular disease, and neuropathy).

Foot sensitivity and adequacy of circulation should be evaluated, and those with impairment should avoid forms of exercise that involve trauma to the feet. Proper foot wear is important.

Table 3.5 Precautions for Patients with Medical Complications

- Insensitive feet or peripheral vascular insufficiency
  - avoid running
  - choose walking, cycling, or swimming
  - emphasize proper footwear
- Untreated or recently treated proliferative retinopathy: avoid exercises associated with:
  - increased intra-abdominal pressure
  - Valsalva-like maneuvers
  - rapid head movements
  - eye trauma
- Hypertension
  - avoid heavy lifting
  - avoid Valsalva-like maneuvers
  - choose exercises that primarily involve the lower-extremity rather than upper-extremity muscle groups

Most patients with active proliferative retinopathy and/or hypertension should avoid strenuous, high-intensity exercises associated with Valsalva-like maneuvers (e.g., weight lifting and certain types of isometrics). Rhythmic exercises involving the lower extremities (e.g., walking, jogging, swimming, and cycling) can potentiate the hypoglycemic effects of both oral medications and insulin. Hypoglycemia can occur during or as much as 12–24 h after the exercise session. SMBG is beneficial in guiding medication adjustments to prevent exercise-induced hypoglycemia. Insulin may need to be decreased on days during which exercise is performed (Table 3.6). This is particularly important if exercise is an adjunct to weight loss. It would be counterproductive to have to treat a hypoglycemic reaction with food or to consume extra food to prevent hypoglycemia in patients on a hypocaloric diet.

Special precautions should be taken when a patient requires or uses drugs that may make him or her more susceptible to exercise-induced hypoglycemia. For example, alcohol and very high doses of salicylates should be avoided because they may themselves produce hypoglycemia. The β-adrenergic-blocking agents may prevent the rapid hepatic glyconeolytic responses that normally correct hypoglycemia. Certain other drugs, including bishydroxycoumarin, phenylbutazone, sulfonamides, and monoamine oxidase inhibitors may potentiate the action of sulfonylureas.

Table 3.6 Guidelines for Safe Exercise

- At all times, patients should carry an identification card and wear a bracelet, necklace, or tag that identifies them as having diabetes.
- If the patient uses insulin:
  - avoid exercise during peak insulin action
  - administer insulin away from working limbs
- If the patient takes single daily dose of intermediate-acting insulin, decrease the dose by as much as 30–35%.
- If the patient uses a combination of short- and intermediate-acting insulin, decrease or omit the short-acting insulin dose and decrease the dose of intermediate-acting insulin by up to 1/3 on days when exercise is planned. This may produce hyperglycemia later in the day that requires a second injection of short-acting insulin.
- If the patient uses only short-acting insulin, reduce the preexercise dose and reduce the postexercise dose based on SMBG. The total dose may need to be reduced by as much as 30–50% on days when exercise is planned.
- Be alert for signs of hypoglycemia during and for several hours after exercise. Have immediate access to a source of readily absorbable carbohydrate (such as glucose tablets) to treat hypoglycemia.
- Take sufficient fluids before, after, and if necessary, during exercise to prevent dehydration.

Patients with type 2 diabetes controlled by diet alone can perform exercise in the same manner as people without diabetes. Supplementary food before, during, or after activity is unnecessary, because hypoglycemia is not a risk.

THE EXERCISE PRESCRIPTION

The key to a successful exercise program is individualization: it must take into account the interests, initial physical condition, and motivation of the patient. A safe exercise prescription requires a complete medical evaluation and specific instructions for managing the exercise program. The patient should start slowly, exercise at regular intervals at least 3–4 times/wk, and gradually increase the duration and intensity of the exercise.

Timing the exercise session in type 2 diabetes may be used advantageously. It appears that exercise performed after 4 PM may reduce hepatic glucose output and decrease fasting glycemia. Exercise after eating may reduce the postprandial hyperglycemia commonly observed in type 2 diabetes. Because exercise is so important, it should be encouraged regardless of when it is performed.

Activity

The type of exercise a patient chooses should be tailored to his or her physical capacity and interests. Most patients can, at a minimum, undertake a walking program safely. Aerobic activities, such as biking, swimming, jogging, and dancing, should be encouraged as well. Biking and swimming are particularly valuable in patients with neuropathy, where foot placement and steady gait may be compromised.

A complete exercise program also includes muscle-strengthening exercises, such as lifting light weights. Armchair exercises can be performed by individuals who are confined to a chair or who may have limited mobility. Flexibility stretches are useful during warm-up and cooldown periods. These not only prepare muscles for an aerobic workout, but also promote improved range of motion, which is especially valuable in elderly people.

Intensity

There are several ways to monitor exercise intensity. One recommendation is to sustain a heart rate at ~60–80% of the maximal heart rate. Generating even 50% of maximum heart rate may be beneficial. Previously sedentary patients should never be given a high-end heart rate goal unless an exercise stress test is performed. However, a low-end heart rate goal, i.e., stay <110 beats/min, can be given without stress testing.

Another alternative is to use a rating of perceived exertion. Patients can be guided to work hard, generally a brisk pace where a light sweat may be present and they perceive they are working. At this pace, they should have enough breath to carry on a conversation. In general, patients should not focus primarily on the intensity of activity, because any activity is preferred to a sedentary lifestyle.

Duration

The vigorous or aerobic portion of an exercise session should last a minimum of 20 min, with a goal of 30–40 min. This should be preceded by a 5- to 10-min warm-up period and followed by a 5- to 10-min cooldown period. These warm-up and cooldown periods may include some weight lifting and flexibility exercises. Most patients will need to work up to this gradually with as little as a 5-min aerobic period that increases incrementally by 1–2 min every 1–2 wk.

Frequency

The benefits of exercise in type 2 diabetes are achieved by repeated bouts of activity <48 h apart. Thus, for fitness, exercise should be performed at least 3 times/wk or every other day. Weight reduction is enhanced by exercise sessions performed 5–6 times/wk.

BIBLIOGRAPHY

American Diabetes Association: Diabetes mellitus and exercise (Position Statement). *Diabetes Care* 16 (Suppl. 2):37, 1993

American Diabetes Association: Exercise and NIDDM (Technical Review). *Diabetes Care* 16 (Suppl. 2):54–58, 1993

Campaigne BN, Lampman RM: *Exercise in the Clinical Management of Diabetes.* Champaign, IL, Human Kinetics, 1994

Hornsby GH, Ed: *Fitness Book for People with Diabetes.* Alexandria, VA, American Diabetes Association, 1994

Gordon NF: *Diabetes: Your Complete Exercise Guide.* Champaign, IL, Human Kinetics, 1993

Graham C, Lasko-McCarthey P: Exercise options for persons with diabetic complications. *Diabetes Educ* 16:212–20, 1990

Maynard T: Physiological response to exercise in diabetes mellitus. *Diabetes Educ* 17:196–206, 1991

Maynard T: Translating the exercise prescription. *Diabetes Educ* 17:384–95, 1991

PHARMACOLOGIC INTERVENTION

The last three years have brought major changes to the pharmacotherapy of type 2 diabetes. Four new classes of oral agents have been approved for use in the United States, and new versions of sulfonylureas and insulin are available. Also, several factors now favor starting pharmacotherapy earlier, when glucose levels are only moderately elevated.

First, the evidence that glycemic control is related to many complications of type 2 diabetes (as well as to those of type 1) is growing stronger. Second, the new definition of diabetes, with fasting plasma glucose (FPG) 126 mg/dl (7 mmol/l) or greater as the main way of making the diagnosis, has focused attention on less severely affected people who have previously not been identified or treated. Third, many of the new oral agents do not cause hypoglycemia when used alone, making early treatment safer. Even so, pharmacologic intervention should only be considered when the person with type 2 diabetes cannot maintain desired levels of glucose control with nutritional measures and regular exercise.

AVAILABLE AGENTS

The agents now available for treating type 2 diabetes are listed in Table 3.7. They may be divided into two categories: those enhancing the effectiveness of insulin, and those augmenting the supply of insulin. The newer agents—metformin, troglitazone, and acarbose—are of the first kind. They have principal actions at the liver, muscle and adipose tissue, and intestinal lumen, respectively, all assisting whatever insulin is available in regulating glucose levels.

Sulfonylureas, repaglinide, and injected insulins are agents of the second kind. Sulfonylureas and repaglinide increase the secretion of insulin into the portal circulation, while injected insulin adds to insulin levels in the systemic circulation. Since the mechanisms of action of all these classes of agents differ, except perhaps in the case of sulfonylureas and repaglinide, they may have complementary or additive effects in many cases.

Agents Enhancing the Effectiveness of Insulin

Since these agents are unlikely to cause hypoglycemia and can be used very early in the natural history of type 2 diabetes, they will be discussed first. Some features of these drugs are shown in Table 3.8.

Metformin. This agent belongs to the biguanide class of drugs. Another biguanide, phenformin, was previously used in the U.S. but was withdrawn because of its tendency to cause lactic acidosis. Metformin is equally effective, but much safer than phenformin. The high-

Table 3.7 Agents Available in the United States

Class	Agent Generic Name	Brand Name
Enhancing the Effects of Insulin		
Biguanide	Metformin	Glucophage
Alpha-glucosidase inhibitor	Acarbose	Precose
Thiazolidinedione	Troglitazone	Rezulin
Augmenting the Supply of Insulin		
Sulfonylurea	Tolbutamide	Orinase
	Chlorpropamide	Diabinese
	Tolazamide	Tolinase
	Glipizide	Glucotrol, Glucotrol XL
	Glyburide	DiaBeta, Micronase, Glynase
	Glimepiride	Amaryl
Meglitinide	Repaglinide	Prandin
Insulin	Human insulin	Humulin, Novolin
	Insulin lispro	Humalog

est concentrations of metformin are found in the gut and liver. It is not metabolized, but is rapidly cleared from plasma by the kidney. Because of rapid clearance, metformin is usually taken 2–3 times daily. Its mechanism of action is complex, probably dominated by reduction of hepatic glucose production at any given level of plasma insulin. It also can improve the response of muscle to insulin (especially at higher dosage), either directly or by reducing calorie intake. Treatment with

Table 3.8 Characteristics of Agents Enhancing the Effects of Insulin

Generic Name	Brand Name	Approved Daily Dosage Range (mg)	Usual Maximum Effective Dosage (mg)	Duration of Action (h)	Clearance
Metformin	Glucophage	500–2,550	1,000 b.i.d.	6–12?	Renal
Acarbose	Precose	25–300	50 t.i.d.	<4	Not absorbed
Troglitazone	Rezulin	200–600	600 once	Weeks	Hepatic

full dosage typically reduces HbA_{1c} by 1–2%. When metformin is started, weight doesn't change or declines slightly, and lipid profiles and blood pressure may improve as well.

The main risk of metformin treatment is lactic acidosis. However, recent experience suggests fatal lactic acidosis associated with metformin is extremely rare, no more common than fatal hypoglycemia associated with sulfonylureas. To minimize this risk, metformin should not be given to patients with significant renal disease (serum creatinine >1.3 for women or >1.5 for men), or to those with serious hepatic or cardiovascular decompensation, and should be used with caution in the elderly. Its main side effects are gastrointestinal, notably anorexia, nausea, or diarrhea. These side effects are frequent (10–30%) at dosages above 1,750 mg daily, but may occur and persist at lower doses in about 5% of patients.

Troglitazone.   Troglitazone is the first thiazolidinedione approved for clinical use in the U.S. It binds to nuclear regulatory sites in muscle and fat cells, directly enhancing insulin's effects on these tissues. It should be taken with food to maximize absorption from the intestine. Its effects develop gradually over several weeks and may take up to 12 wk to reach a peak. In people without diabetes with poor tissue-responses to insulin (insulin resistance), it reduces insulin levels in plasma and may reduce triglycerides and increase HDL levels. In people with impaired glucose tolerance, it improves glucose tolerance as well as reduces insulin levels. Patients with overt type 2 diabetes have varying reductions of insulin and glucose levels with troglitazone. Studies of Japanese and European patients, who are less obese and probably less insulin resistant than patients in the U.S., show smaller reductions of HbA_{1c} (0.5–1.0%) with troglitazone than are typically seen with metformin (1–2%) when these agents are used alone. Studies in the U.S. that selected more obese patients showed greater reductions in HbA_{1c} with troglitazone, especially when it was added to insulin or a sulfonylurea.

Fluid retention and weight gain have been the main adverse events in human trials of troglitazone. However, cardiac changes in animal studies of related drugs have led to the recommendation that troglitazone be used cautiously in patients with heart disease. Its favorable effects on insulin resistance and lipoprotein patterns suggest long-term cardiovascular benefits, but this hypothesis has not been directly tested. Small increases of liver enzyme levels may occur, and a few cases of severe liver disease have been reported. Troglitazone should be used cautiously in patients with liver disease. In all patients, liver enzyme levels should be measured before starting treatment; every mo for 6 mo, then every other mo for the first yr; and periodically thereafter. The drug should be discontinued if significant abnormalities appear.

Acarbose.   Acarbose is the first α-glucosidase inhibitor to come to clinical use. Its action occurs in the intestinal lumen, where it competitively inhibits enzymes that split polysaccharides into simple sugars. Its main effect is on starches, but cleavage of the disaccharide sucrose to glucose and fructose is also reduced. Cleavage of lactose is unaffected. The result of this action is to delay absorption of dietary carbohydrates until they have passed to the mid or distal small bowel, so that postprandial peaks of plasma glucose are blunted. To achieve this effect, acarbose tablets must be taken at the beginning of meals. In studies of large European and Canadian populations, acarbose reduced HbA$_{1c}$ by 0.5–1.0%. In theory, its power should be greater in groups of patients with especially prominent postprandial hyperglycemia, but studies to confirm this are lacking.

Very little acarbose is absorbed from the intestine, but liver enzyme changes have occurred in a few cases. Its main adverse effects are flatulence, abdominal distress or distension, and diarrhea. These result from excessive blockade of carbohydrate absorption in the small bowel, leading to fermentation and gas production in the colon. They are minimized by low initial dosage with gradual titration upward. Intestinal distension or diarrhea may be harmful in the presence of inflammatory bowel disease or other major intestinal disorders.

Agents Augmenting the Supply of Insulin

Sulfonylureas.   These agents are only effective in the presence of endogenous insulin. Therefore, their main effect must be at the β-cell where they bind to the potassium channel complex on the surface membrane. When given initially, they sharply increase insulin secretion and reduce daytime plasma glucose, sometimes to hypoglycemic levels. Used chronically, individual doses have less immediate effect, and the overall pattern shows reduction of fasting and 24-h mean glucose with little reduction of postprandial increments. Physiologically, their main effect is to reduce overnight hepatic glucose production by enhancing insulin secretion.

Whether sulfonylureas have significant effects beyond the β-cell has been debated. After chronic sulfonylurea treatment the peripheral tissues may become more sensitive to insulin, but this seems largely due to waning of the adverse effects of hyperglycemia (glucotoxicity). Sulfonylureas bind to potassium channels in various tissues, including vascular tissue, and may reduce vasodilation in response to tissue injury. Whether this effect is clinically important is unknown, but it may relate to the concerns about cardiovascular risks of sulfonylureas raised in 1970 when the University Group Diabetes Program (UGDP) study was published. These concerns have diminished because there is no agreement on interpretation of data from that study, and similar studies could not confirm its findings. A common interpretation has been that any small cardiovascular risk that might accompany sulfonylurea treatment is obscured by the major metabolic benefits of effective treatment.

The main complication of sulfonylurea treatment is hypoglycemia. Elderly patients are more susceptible, especially when they have declining renal function or tend to skip meals. Side effects are uncommon, but the leading ones are gastrointestinal symptoms, such as nausea and vomiting, and skin reactions, including rashes, purpura, and pruritis. Other side effects include hematologic reactions (leukopenia, thrombocytopenia, or hemolytic anemia) and cholestasis (with or without jaundice). Modest weight gain may occur when treatment is started.

Some features of the sulfonylureas now available in the United States are shown in Table 3.9. When taken at maximally effective dosage, they all have equal ability to reduce hyperglycemia, equivalent to 1–2% HbA$_{1c}$. They differ in other ways. The first-generation sulfonylureas (tolbuta-

Table 3.9 Characteristics of Sulfonylureas

Generic Name	Brand Name	Approved Daily Dosage Range (mg)	Near Maximum Effective Dosage (mg)	Duration of Action (h)	Clearance
Tolbutamide	Orinase	500–3,000	1,000 t.i.d.	6–12	Hepatic
Chlorpropamide	Diabinese	100–500	500 once	>48	Renal
Tolazamide	Tolinase	100–1,000	500 b.i.d.	12–24	Hepatic, renal
Glipizide	Glucotrol	2.5–40	10 b.i.d.	12–18	Hepatic
Glipizide (extended release)	Glucotrol XL	5–10	10 once	24	Hepatic
Glyburide	DiaBeta	1.25–20	5 b.i.d.	12–24	Hepatic
	Micronase	1.25–2	5 b.i.d.	12–24	Hepatic, renal
	Glynase	0.75–12	3 b.i.d.	12–24	Hepatic, renal
Glimepiride	Amaryl	1–8	4 once	24	Hepatic or renal
Repaglinide	Prandin	1–16	4 t.i.d.	2–6	Hepatic

mide, tolazamide, and chlorpropamide) bind significantly to plasma proteins and have high milligram dosage requirements. Because of the protein binding, they can displace or be displaced by other agents, such as salicylates or warfarin, leading to drug interactions. Tolbutamide is rapidly cleared by the liver and must be taken 2–3 times daily. Chlorpropamide is slowly cleared by the kidney and accumulates when renal function declines, and it may cause serious hypoglycemia when this happens. Chlorpropamide also may cause an antabuse-like intolerance to alcohol, or potentiate antidiuretic hormone action leading to water intoxication. Because of these limitations, use of these agents is declining.

The second-generation sulfonylureas (glyburide and glipizide) are largely free of interactions with other drugs and have lower total dosage requirements. Both are metabolized mainly by the liver, but renal insufficiency can enhance their ability to cause hypoglycemia. Declining renal function is especially problematic in the case of glyburide, which has an active metabolite that must be excreted by the kidney. Both require twice-daily dosage for full effect.

The newest sulfonylurea preparations are extended-release glipizide and glimepiride. Extended-release formulation of glipizide achieves a 24-h effect for a drug that ordinarily has a much shorter duration. Glimepiride is a new sulfonylurea that is slowly cleared by the liver. Like cholorpropamide, both are fully effective when taken once daily, but they are less likely to cause hypoglycemia. Glimepiride and its only active metabolite are both cleared by the liver, so renal insufficiency should alter its effect only slightly. Maximal effect of extended-release glipizide is reached with 10 mg once daily, and of glimepiride with 4 mg once daily.

Repaglinide.   This new agent has just been introduced into use. Although structurally different from the sulfonylureas, it also binds to the potassium channel complex on the β-cell and enhances the release of insulin. It is rapidly absorbed after oral administration and rapidly cleared by hepatic metabolism. This rapid time-course of action calls for two or three doses daily with meals. Studies available at this time suggest that repaglinide reduces HbA_{1c} just as well as sulfonylureas but has slightly greater effect on postprandial glycemia and slightly less effect on overnight fasting glycemia. No important side effects other than hypoglycemia have been identified. Whether there are clinically significant differences between repaglinide and sulfonylureas in mechanism of action or tendency to cause hypoglycemia is currently under study.

INSULINS

Although insulin has been used therapeutically for over 70 years, some aspects of its use are new. Insulins extracted from the pancreases of cattle and pigs are no longer widely used. They have largely been replaced by insulin that is synthesized by genetically altered microorganisms, and that is structurally identical to human insulin. The familiar extended-action preparations are still available, as shown in Table 3.10, but they are all slightly quicker and shorter acting when made from human rather than animal insulin. This difference is less apparent in treatment of type 2 diabetes than with type 1 diabetes, because absorption of insulin after subcutaneous injection is generally slower in older, more obese type 2 patients than in younger, physically active type 1 patients.

The first structurally modified variant of human insulin, insulin lispro, recently came into use. This insulin analog differs from human insulin in having the order of two amino acids, lysine and proline, reversed at one site. This small modification reduces the tendency of insulin in a vial to aggregate into dimers and hexamers that delays absorption of unmodified insulins after subcutaneous injection. Insulin lispro is absorbed almost as rapidly as insulin is normally secreted after a meal, so the postprandial insulin pattern resembles that in people without diabetes. Thus, better postprandial glycemic control is possible. Insulin lispro should be taken immediately (<5 min) before a meal, which many patients find more convenient than waiting 15–45 min for the meal after insulin injection, as is desired with regular insulin. Other than hypoglycemia with unskillful use, no significant adverse effects of insulin lispro have been identified. Whether insulin lispro is safer or

Table 3.10 Characteristics of Human Insulins and Lispro

Preparation	Timing of Action		
	Onset	Peak	Duration
Short-acting			
Lispro	5 min	0.5–1 h	3 h
Regular	30 min	2–5 h	5–8 h
Intermediate-acting			
NPH	1–2 h	6–10 h	16–20 h
Lente	1–2 h	8–12 h	18–24 h
Long-acting			
Ultralente	4–6 h	10–18 h	24–28 h
Mixtures			
70/30, 50/50	30 min	7–12 h	16–4 h

This table summarizes the typical time course of various insulin preparations. These values are highly variable among individuals. Even in a given person, these values vary depending on the site and depth of injection, skin temperature, and exercise.

more effective than regular insulin in controlling 24-h glucose and HbA$_{1c}$ in type 2 diabetes has not been determined.

Premixed combinations of insulins are now in wide use. The forms available in the United States are 70/30 (70% NPH and 30% regular) and 50/50 (50% NPH and 50% regular) insulins. These fixed combinations have serious limitations for patients with type 1 diabetes, who need to modify insulin doses and ratios very frequently. In contrast, many patients with type 2 diabetes have substantial endogenous insulin and can use premixed insulin both conveniently, with less time spent preparing the dose, and effectively, with good glycemic results.

Insulin has essentially unlimited power to reduce plasma glucose. It reduces the blood glucose level by suppressing hepatic glucose production and by increasing glucose uptake by insulin-sensitive tissues, notably muscle and adipose tissue. As with sulfonylureas, the improved glycemic control achieved with insulin therapy generally increases the responsiveness of tissues to insulin. The main practical limitation in achieving treatment objectives with insulin is the risk of hypoglycemia. Also, patients with type 2 diabetes, who are typically already obese, usually gain weight when insulin treatment is started. Other side effects include immediate skin reactions at injection sites (itching, redness, and swelling), or persistent lumps or swelling at these sites that may represent delayed hypersensitivity reactions. These allergy-related problems are less common with current insulin preparations than with previous ones, and may be less common in people with type 2 diabetes than in those with type 1 diabetes.

SELECTING AN AGENT TO BEGIN TREATMENT

With more agents to choose from, pharmacotherapy of type 2 diabetes has become both more effective and more complex. Different agents have different clinical effects (Table 3.11). The first treatment decision is required when a patient is found, despite the best possible

Table 3.11 Comparison of the Clinical Effects of Oral Agents

Agent	Site of Action	Effect on Glucose	HbA$_{1c}$ Reduction (%)
Acarbose	Small intestine	⇓ postprandial increase	0.5–1
Metformin	Liver, muscle	⇓ fasting and 24-h mean	1–2
Repaglinide	β-cell	⇓ fasting and postprandial	1–2
Sulfonylureas	β-cell	⇓ fasting and 24-h mean	1–2
Troglitazone	Muscle, fat	⇓ fasting and postprandial	0.5–1.5

effort with lifestyle modification, to have HbA$_{1c}$ >7%. The epidemiologic evidence now available justifies starting pharmacologic treatment at this level of control, although physicians may in some cases prefer rededication to lifestyle efforts until HbA$_{1c}$ reaches 7.5 or 8%. The choice of agent depends, in part, on the level of control at which treatment is started.

Fasting Plasma Glucose 126–140 mg/dl

Patients with HbA$_{1c}$ above 7% but relatively modest elevations of FPG are candidates for one of the three agents that do not cause hypoglycemia when used alone: metformin, troglitazone, or acarbose. Fasting plasma glucose in the 126–140 mg/dl range defines this situation. This corresponds to fasting capillary blood glucose (measured by most available glucose meters) in the 110–125 mg/dl range. Each agent may be especially effective for certain groups of patients. Metformin mainly reduces FPG rather than postprandial increases, and it is effective for both obese and nonobese patients. Troglitazone is most effective for very insulin-resistant patients, who can most readily be identified by central obesity. Acarbose mainly reduces postprandial increases of glucose, and it is most suited to patients for whom this is a leading problem. All three agents are powerful enough to reduce glucose and HbA$_{1c}$ to target levels in this setting.

The adverse effects of each agent should be considered before starting treatment. Metformin should not be used for patients with hepatic or renal insufficiency. Troglitazone should not be given to those with serious cardiac or hepatic disease. Acarbose should be avoided when the patient has serious intestinal or liver disease.

In each case, the dosage should be started low and titrated upward slowly. The starting dose of metformin is 500 mg 1–2 times daily with breakfast and/or the evening meal. After 2–4 wk, dosage may be increased to 500 mg 3–4 times daily or 850 mg 2–3 times daily. The starting dose of troglitazone is 200 mg daily, taken with any meal, with increases to 300, 400, or 600 mg if necessary. Because the onset of action is slow, dosage generally should not be increased more often than every 2 mo. Acarbose is best started at 25 mg once daily, and increased incrementally every 2 wk to a maximum of 50–100 mg with each meal (maximum 50 mg t.i.d. if body wt <60 kg).

Fasting Plasma Glucose >140 mg/dl

When FPG is >140 mg/dl, sulfonylureas may be added to the list of options. This level corresponds to fasting capillary blood glucose >125 mg/dl. Most patients will respond to a sulfonylurea. However, patients with renal insufficiency are not good candidates because of increased risk of hypoglycemia. Dosage should be started low unless

FPG is >250 mg/dl. Typical starting doses are 2.5 mg glyburide, 5 mg glipizide, or 1 mg glimepiride. Dosage may be increased at any time, since therapeutic effects are apparent within days, and side effects other than hypoglycemia are not generally dose-related. Maximal clinical effectiveness is usually reached with 10 mg glyburide or 10 mg standard glipizide twice daily, or 10 mg extended-release glipizide or 4 mg glimepiride once daily. Some of these doses are lower than the maximum recommended doses.

Insulin may also be used for initial treatment of type 2 diabetes, although most patients prefer to use oral treatments first. Initiation of insulin treatment will be described later in this chapter.

PRIMARY AND SECONDARY FAILURE OF TREATMENTS

In some cases, a treatment may fail when first tried. This has been called primary failure, and in some cases it indicates incorrect selection of the treatment. For example, a sulfonylurea will not work for a patient with type 1 diabetes and no endogenous insulin. Insulin treatment is required from the start in such patients. Similarly, troglitazone is unlikely to improve glycemic control when insulin resistance is lacking. In other cases, the agent may be appropriately selected but not powerful enough. When initial glucose levels are very high, a given agent may have its expected effect but still lack the power required to achieve target levels of control. This is common when FPG is well over 200 mg/dl and HbA_{1c} over 10% when an oral agent is started. Either a sulfonylurea or metformin would be expected to reduce FPG by 50–80 mg/dl, and HbA_{1c} by 1–2%. Some patients will have exceptional responses, but most will not achieve HbA_{1c} values close to 7%. Adding a second agent to the first one (combined or combination therapy) may be necessary to reach target levels.

Even when effective at first, all therapies for type 2 diabetes become less effective over time. This applies even to lifestyle changes and insulin. Secondary failure of treatments is related to progression of the underlying abnormalities of the β-cell and insulin action. The United Kingdom Prospective Diabetes Study has shown that, on continuous treatment, HbA_{1c} increases at a rate averaging 0.2% yearly or 1% over 5 yr. Thus, a treatment successfully reducing HbA_{1c} from 7.5 to 6.5% is likely to show secondary failure, defined as a return to the initial level of control, within 5 yr. Substituting another oral agent for the one no longer fully effective is rarely helpful in this situation.

Oral Combinations

Combinations of agents may achieve or restore glycemic control after primary or secondary failure of monotherapy, postponing the need for insulin treatment. The best-tested combinations of oral agents are sulfonylurea with metformin and sulfonylurea with acarbose. However, other combinations are possible, and owing to the different mechanisms of action of the agents, the therapeutic effects should be additive in most cases. Fortunately, the side effects of the various agents (except for hypoglycemia) have not been shown to be additive.

Since both insulin deficiency and reduced insulin action contribute to hyperglycemia in most cases, combinations of a sulfonylurea with one or more of the other agents are most logical. A patient started with a sulfonylurea may have metformin, troglitazone, or acarbose added. A patient started with one of the agents aiding insulin action will usually benefit from addition of a sulfonylurea. Three-drug oral combinations have not been well studied, but may be effective for some patients. Eventually, secondary failure of oral combinations will occur.

STARTING INSULIN THERAPY

Insulin is capable of restoring glycemia to near normal in most patients with type 2 diabetes. Although this therapy may result in elevated insulin levels, the relationship, if any, between hyperinsulinemia caused by insulin treatment and the long-term complications of diabetes is unknown. In contrast, there is clear evidence that hyperglycemia worsens the complications. Therefore, the focus should be on glucose control rather than on the theoretical deleterious effects of hyperinsulinemia.

Some physicians prefer insulin to oral hypoglycemic agents as the primary pharmacologic intervention, after diet and exercise are no longer successful alone. Insulin is particularly appropriate as primary therapy for patients with rapid uncontrolled weight loss unexplained by diet who also have severe hyperglycemia, especially when accompanied by ketonemia and/or ketonuria. Such patients may be severely insulin deficient and, in fact, have late-onset type 1 rather than type 2 diabetes. Late-onset type 1 diabetes is more common than previously recognized, and may account for 10% of cases of diabetes diagnosed in adults.

Other indications for the use of insulin include:

- periods of acute injury, stress, infection, surgery, or glucocorticoid treatment
- pregnancy
- renal or hepatic disease or allergies that preclude use of oral therapies
- primary or secondary failure of oral agents

Note that any metabolic state or drug that increases the requirement for insulin or interferes with insulin secretion may require temporary insulin therapy. Management with insulin during pregnancy or surgery is discussed on pages 73–75. Insulin therapy should be used with particular care in poorly adherent patients who are unwilling or unable to perform SMBG, or patients for whom hypoglycemia is a serious risk, such as those with cerebrovascular disease or unstable angina.

Because the tissues of patients with type 2 diabetes are usually less responsive to insulin, large doses of insulin may be necessary. This is particularly true for severely obese patients with type 2 diabetes, who may require 100 to 200 U daily or more. More than one daily injection is usually required. Most often, a mixture of short and intermediate-acting insulins given twice daily will be effective. Beginning to use insulin is a milestone in a person's experience. It requires education and emotional support, and more careful monitoring of glucose because of the possibility of hypoglycemia. The tactics for starting insulin may vary somewhat, depending on whether oral agents are already being used.

Insulin without Oral Agents

When insulin is started by patients not taking oral agents, a single injection of intermediate-acting insulin may be given either before breakfast or at bedtime. Patients with predominantly daytime hyperglycemia are likely to respond better to a morning injection, and those with marked fasting hyperglycemia may be candidates for a bedtime injection. A conservative starting dose of 10 U is unlikely to cause hypoglycemia, yet will improve glycemia somewhat while the patient is learning to handle and inject insulin. Glucose monitoring by SMBG should be done at least twice daily, with tests before breakfast and the evening meal to assess the response (Table 3.12). Some patients will have excellent responses with a single injection and may maintain target levels of control this way for some time. In other cases, two daily injections will be required for best results. Generally, a mixture of intermediate and short-acting insulins should be given before breakfast and before the evening meal. The ratio of the morning to evening doses needed varies among patients. Some need up to 2/3 of the total in the morning, others 2/3 in the evening, and many need approximately equal amounts at each injection. The same is true of the ratio of intermediate to short-acting insulin at each dose. Some patients do very well with a 2-to-1 ratio; others do better with a 1-to-1 ratio. A simple and reasonable way to begin two-injection treatment is with 10 U of premixed 70/30 insulin (70% NPH, 30% regular) twice daily. Both the dosage and distribution should be modified as indicated by the SMBG results. Relatively nonobese patients may achieve good glucose control with no more than 20–40 U daily. More obese patients will need more, often 100–200 U daily. Many patients will need to mix intermediate and short-acting insulins from separate vials, in order to vary the ratio for optimal results.

Table 3.12 Insulin Regimen and Timing of Self-Monitoring of Blood Glucose

Insulin	Time Injected	Period of Greatest Activity	SMBG Reflecting Insulin Action
Short-acting	Before a meal	Between that meal and the next meal or bedtime	Both 1-2 h after the meal and just before the next meal
Intermediate-acting	Before breakfast	Between lunch and evening meal	Before evening meal
	Before evening meal	Between midnight and breakfast	Before breakfast
	At bedtime	Between 4 AM and breakfast	Before breakfast
Long-acting	Before breakfast or bedtime	Mostly overnight, because short-acting insulin overrides its effect during the day	Before breakfast

Adapted from Davidson MB: How to get the most out of insulin therapy. *Clinical Diabetes* 8:65–73, 1990.

Insulin After Failure of Oral Agents

The task of starting insulin is slightly different when oral agents, have been used previously and secondary failure has ensued. There are two options. The first, and traditional, option is to stop oral agents and begin insulin alone. However, after secondary failure of oral agents, insulin must be used more aggressively than when it is the initial treatment. The reason for this is that by the time secondary failure of oral agents has occurred, the underlying defects of insulin secretion and action have progressed, and withdrawing oral agents may lead to rapid loss of glycemic control. A single injection of insulin is unlikely to be effective, and two injections should be started immediately, at a dosage of 10–15 U twice daily. The dosage should be increased at frequent intervals, such as every 2–3 days, guided by the results of SMBG.

Alternatively, a simpler method may be used. A bedtime injection of intermediate or long-acting insulin (or 70/30 insulin before the evening meal for obese patients) may be added while oral therapy is continued. The rationale is that supplementing with overnight insulin will control fasting hyperglycemia, while continuing the oral agents will prevent worsening of glycemic control during the time that the insulin dosage is titrated upward. In addition, beginning evening insulin while continuing oral agents causes less hyperinsulinemia and weight gain than starting multiple injections of insulin alone. Treatment can begin with 10 U, and the dosage may be increased by 5- to 10-U increments weekly. When fasting SMBG values reach 120 mg/dl, FPG will be ~140 mg/dl. As with other treatments, secondary failure will occur eventually, shown by increased afternoon glucose values and rising HbA_{1c}. Two injections of insulin, usually before breakfast and the evening meal, are then required.

LONG-TERM COMBINATIONS OF ORAL AGENTS WITH INSULIN

By the time two daily injections are needed, β-cell function has usually declined enough that sulfonylureas provide little benefit and should be stopped. Whether the insulin-enhancing oral agents continue to be helpful and should be continued has not been well studied. In theory, reduction of insulin resistance (by troglitazone), limitation of weight gain (by metformin), and improvement of lipids (by either) may reduce vascular risks. Certainly these agents can reduce the total insulin dosage, sometimes preventing the need to use more than a single 100-U syringeful at a given time of day. For these reasons, continuing the agents enhancing insulin action may be given serious consideration.

The effect of combining metformin, acarbose, or troglitazone with insulin is best seen when one of these agents is added to previously established insulin treatment. When either metformin or troglitazone is added to insulin therapy of obese, insulin-resistant people, up to a 50% reduction of insulin dosage may be possible while glycemic control remains the same or improves. In a few cases, insulin can be discontinued entirely while a combination of oral agents is used to maintain control, but this not the main reason to consider adding an insulin-enhancing agent. The main purpose is to restore glucose control to target levels.

ADJUSTING INSULIN DOSAGE IN LONG-TERM TYPE 2 DIABETES

By 15–20 yr after the onset of type 2 diabetes, many patients will have markedly reduced endogenous insulin secretion. At this time, glycemic variability increases and reliance on injected insulin becomes greater. Therefore, treatment of these patients becomes more like that of type 1 diabetes than it was earlier in the course of their type 2 diabetes. Both the patient and the physician must be aware of the time course of action of the various kinds of insulin and the times at which hypoglycemia is most likely to occur. Blood glucose levels must be monitored at home

Table 3.13 Sample Insulin Regimens for Achieving Glycemic Control

Regimen	Before Breakfast	Before Lunch	Before Evening Meal	Bedtime
1	Intermediate-acting + Short-acting		Intermediate-acting + Short-acting	
2	Intermediate-acting + Short-acting		Short-acting	Intermediate-acting
3	Intermediate-acting + Short-acting	Short-acting	Short-acting	Intermediate-acting
4	Short-acting	Short-acting	Short-acting	Long-acting

regularly by the patient or a responsible helper, and adjustments of meal pattern and/or insulin made when necessary.

Table 3.12 shows the times at which different kinds of injected insulin are most active in reducing glucose levels when given at various times of day. Short-acting insulin is given before meals and is active during the interval up to 3 h after the meal (in the case of lispro) and 6 or more h after the meal (in the case of regular insulin). Intermediate-acting insulin has peak activity 6–12 h after injection. Since intermediate-acting insulin is commonly given before breakfast, before the evening meal, or at bedtime, it may cause hypoglycemia in the late afternoon, from midnight to 4 AM, or just before breakfast.

Four different insulin regimens are shown in Table 3.13. Regimen 1 is the two-injection regimen using both intermediate-acting and short-acting insulin described previously. It is effective for many patients with type 2 diabetes as long as they retain significant endogenous insulin. The dosages used at each injection can be adjusted on the basis of SMBG results. Disproportionately high values before lunch suggest inadequate short-acting insulin in the morning injection, and high values at bedtime suggest the short-acting insulin before the evening meal is insufficient. Similarly, high glucose readings before the evening meal or breakfast suggest the need to increase the morning or evening intermediate-acting dose, respectively. Low glucose values suggest excessive dosage of the insulins responsible for coverage at each of these times of day. When adjustments of individual components of the insulin regimen are necessary, premixed insulins (70/30 or 50/50) are less effective, and better results will be obtained if the patient mixes the insulins for each injection.

Regimen 2 differs from Regimen 1 in that the evening meal intermediate-acting insulin has been moved to bedtime. The advantage of this change is to reduce the chance of hypoglycemia between midnight and 4 AM by shifting the peak effect of the dose closer to breakfast. This change is necessary mostly for active, less obese patients who absorb insulins rapidly and may develop nocturnal hypoglycemia on the two-injection regimen.

Regimen 3 may be desirable for patients who tend to have widely variable SMBG readings in the late afternoon when using Regimen 2. Moving part of the short-acting dose given at breakfast to lunchtime generally smooths afternoon control. Regimen 4 is a full basal-bolus regimen of the kind commonly used for type 1 diabetes. The long-acting dose is meant to provide basal insulin levels over 24 h, and it can be given at breakfast or the evening meal instead of bedtime in some patients, or it can be split into smaller doses and given twice daily. This regimen may allow greater flexibility with eating and exercise patterns. Individualized regimens may be required as determined by meal patterns or by SMBG results. For example, some older people awaken late and eat just two meals, the first (and sometimes main) meal close to midday and a second meal in the evening. In this case, the first insulin injection may best be given before the midday meal and the second before the evening meal.

BIBLIOGRAPHY

American Diabetes Association: Insulin administration (Position Statement). *Diabetes Care* 20 (Suppl. 1):S46–49, 1997

Bell PM, Hadden DR: Metformin. *Endocrinol Metab Clin North Am* 26:523–37, 1997

Burge MR, Schade DS: Insulins. *Endocrinol Metab Clin North Am* 26:575–98, 1997

DeFronzo RA, Goodman AM, the Multicenter Metformin Study Group: Efficacy of metformin in patients with non-insulin-dependent diabetes mellitus. *N Engl J Med* 333:541–49, 1995

Edelman SV, Henry RR: Intensive insulin therapy for patients with type II diabetes. In *Diabetes Mellitus: A Fundamental and Clinical Text.* LeRoith D, Taylor SI, Olefsky JM, Eds. Philadelphia, Lippincott-Raven, 1996, pp. 647–60

Garber AJ, Duncan TG, Goodman AM, Mills DJ, Rohlf JL: Efficacy of metformin in type 2 diabetes; results of a double-blind, placebo-controlled, dose-response trial. *Am J Med* 103:491–97, 1997

Goldberg RB, Holvey SM, Schneider J, the Glimepiride Study Group: A dose-response study of glimepiride in patients with NIDDM who have previously received sulfonylurea agents. *Diabetes Care* 19:849–56, 1996

Henry RR: Thiazolidinediones. *Endocrinol Metab Clin North Am* 26:553–73, 1997

Herrmann LS, Schersten B, Bitzen P-O, Kjellstrom T, Lindgarde F, Melander A: Therapeutic comparison of metformin and sulfonylurea, alone and in various combinations. *Diabetes Care* 20:1100–1109, 1997

Inzucchi SE, Maggs DG, Spollett GR, Page SL, Rife FS, Walton V, Shulman GI. Efficacy and metabolic effects of metformin and troglitazone in type 2 diabetes mellitus, *N Engl J Med* 338:67–72, 1998

Lebovitz HE: Alpha-glucosidase inhibitors. *Endocrinol Metab Clin North Am* 26:539–51, 1997

Misbin RI, Green L, Stadel BU, Gweriguian JL, Gubbi A, Flemming GA: Lactic acidosis in patients with diabetes treated with metformin. *N Engl J Med* 338:265–66, 1998

Schwartz S, Raskin P, Fonseca U, Graveline JF, Effect of troglitazone in insulin-treated patients with type 2 diabetes. *N Engl J Med* 338:861–66, 1998

Shank ML, DelPrato S, DeFronzo RA: Bedtime insulin/daytime glipizide: effective therapy for sulfonylurea failures in NIDDM. *Diabetes* 44:165–72, 1995

Simonsen DC, Kourides IA, Feinglos M, Shamoon H, Fischette CT, the Glipizide Gastrointestinal System Study Group: Efficacy, safety, and dose-response characteristics of glipizide gastrointestinal therapeutic system on glycemic control and insulin secretion in NIDDM. *Diabetes Care* 20:597–606, 1997

U.K. Prospective Diabetes Study 16: Overview of 6 years' therapy of type II diabetes: a progressive disease. *Diabetes* 44:1249–58, 1995

Wolffenbuttel BHR, Nijst L., Sels JPJE, Menheere PPCA, Muller PG, Nieuwenhuijzen S, Kruseman AC: Effects of a new oral hypoglycemic agent, repaglinide, on metabolic control in sulfonylurea-treated patients with NIDDM. *Eur J Clin Pharmacol* 45:113–116, 1993

Zimmerman BR: Sulfonylureas. *Endocrinol Metab Clin North Am* 26:511–22, 1997

SPECIAL THERAPEUTIC PROBLEMS

Pregnancy and surgery in patients with diabetes are complicating situations that require extraordinary care to protect the patient against additional problems.

PREGNANCY

Pregnancy can cause clinical difficulties for both the patient and her unborn baby. The infant of a mother with diabetes has an increased risk of death, prematurity, and morbidity (congenital defects, macrosomia, hypoglycemia, hypocalcemia, hyperbilirubinemia, and respiratory distress syndrome). The mother with diabetes faces an increased risk of acceleration of microvascular complications involving the kidneys and eyes, particularly if hypertension is present.

In a patient with diabetes, pregnancy should be planned so that conception occurs when the patient has near-normal fasting, preprandial, and postprandial plasma glucose levels and HbA_{1c} values within the goal range. After conception, treatment should not only continue to achieve glycemic goals, but also meet the nutritional requirements of the fetus. The patient who is treated with oral diabetes medications should be switched to insulin therapy before conception. If the patient is being treated with oral diabetes agents and she becomes pregnant, she should be switched to insulin.

The physician should inform the patient of the risks to her and the baby. Because the risks of pregnancy in association with diabetes mellitus are great and involve both mother and fetus/newborn, and the treatment program (multiple injections of insulin or use of the insulin pump and euglycemic regulation) is complex, the care of a pregnant woman with diabetes should involve appropriate specialists. Consultation with a physician skilled in the care of pregnant women with diabetes should be sought before conception or as soon as pregnancy is diagnosed to effect normalization of blood glucose levels.

Goals for glycemic control in diabetic women during pregnancy are:

- fasting: 60–90 mg/dl (3.3–5.0 mmol/l)
- premeal: 60–105 mg/dl (3.3–5.8 mmol/l)
- 1-h postprandial: 110–130 mg/dl (6.1–7.3 mmol/l)
- 2-h postprandial: 90–120 mg/dl (5.0–6.7 mmol/l)
- 0200–0600: 60–120 mg/dl (3.3–6.7 mmol/l)

The care of a pregnant woman with diabetes requires a skilled health care team. The physician who assumes responsibility for such a patient must be completely familiar with proper management of the patient and her fetus/newborn during pregnancy, just before and during delivery, and immediately after delivery. The same vigorous attention to glycemic regulation and proper management of the patient and her fetus/newborn must be given to the individual who develops gestational diabetes during the second or third trimester.

SURGERY

It is now possible for a patient with diabetes mellitus to undergo surgical operations with little more than normal risk, unless the operation is done under emergency conditions that do not allow complete evaluation and preparation of the patient. Proper surgical management of the patient should be of concern to the physician in charge of the patient with type 2 diabetes mellitus. Conditions requiring surgery often develop in older people in general, and in patients with diabetes in particular (e.g., occlusive vascular disease, gallbladder disease, or cataracts).

Unless the surgical condition is an emergency, the patient should be allowed sufficient time to achieve acceptable control of hyperglycemia before surgery. If possible, the patient should have a complete evaluation of metabolic state and thorough assessment of diabetic complications, including renal and cardiovascular disease, before surgery.

The objectives of management before, during, and after surgery are to prevent hypoglycemia, which can lead to coma, and to prevent excessive hyperglycemia and ketoacidosis, which can complicate postoperative care by causing dehydration, excessive protein loss, and electrolyte imbalance. To accomplish these ends, the anesthetic technique (regional or general) and the anesthetic agent should disrupt metabolic control as little as possible. Special attention should be given to maintaining proper fluid and electrolyte balance and blood glucose levels. Patients with diabetes who have been treated with diet or oral agents may need insulin therapy for control of hyperglycemia during the acute stress period of a major surgical procedure.

More authorities have begun to advocate intravenous infusion of insulin instead of subcutaneous administration. Intravenous administration circumvents problems of insulin delivery in the event of peripheral shutdown (hypotension and/or shock), which might occur during major surgery. Furthermore, intravenous administration makes it possible to carefully control the amount and speed of insulin delivery appropriately based on frequent measurement of blood glucose.

With either administration technique, the operative team should understand the management objectives and work together to achieve them. In this critical effort, it is particularly important to involve an anesthesiologist who is trained in the management of patients with diabetes.

To assume responsibility for the management of patients with type 2 diabetes during and after surgical procedures, the clinician must learn specific techniques involved in preparing the patient for surgery and for managing the patient during and after the operation. The major principles governing the management of surgical candidates on the day of operation are presented in Table 3.14.

Table 3.14 Major Principles Governing Management of Patients with Diabetes During Surgery in Hospitals and Ambulatory Care Centers

- General management goals are to control hyperglycemia to a degree so as to prevent hypoglycemia and ketoacidosis. Short-term modest hyperglycemia is preferred over attempts at euglycemia with its attendant risk for hypoglycemia.
- Management is considered satisfactory when random plasma glucose levels during and after surgery are between 125–200 mg/dl (6.9–11.1 mmol/l). The clinician in charge must make judgments about target plasma glucose levels, taking into consideration the skill and availability of the operative/postoperative team.
- Plasma glucose levels should be determined frequently in the perioperative period as a guide to therapy; urine glucose levels are unreliable. The usual recommendation is to obtain plasma glucose levels every 4–6 h until the patient resumes oral feeding, unless severe hyperglycemia necessitates more intense management. The patient whose concurrent illness renders him or her unstable metabolically because of the use of glucocorticoids or enteral or parenteral nutrition may best be controlled with an intravenous insulin infusion.
- Mild hyperglycemia is preferable to hypoglycemia, especially during surgery. The actual amount of insulin used is determined by considering the patient's plasma glucose levels before, during, and after surgery, and, in the case of an insulin-taking patient, the usual insulin requirement. Preoperative doses of insulin may be:
  - the usual dose of intermediate-acting insulin, which necessitates i.v. glucose continuously
  - half the dose of intermediate-acting insulin, often with a small amount of rapid-acting insulin added to glucose-containing i.v. solutions
  - no intermediate-acting insulin, which necessitates short-acting insulin added to i.v. solutions

---

BIBLIOGRAPHY

Alberti KGMM: Diabetes and surgery. In *Diabetes Mellitus: Theory and Practice*. Fourth ed. Rifkin H, Porte D, Eds. New York, Elsevier, 1990, pp. 626–33

Arauz-Pacheco C, Raskin P: *Therapy for Diabetes Mellitus and Related Disorders*. Second ed. Lebovitz HE, Ed. Alexandria, VA, American Diabetes Association, 1994, pp. 156–63

Jovanovic-Peterson L, Ed. *Medical Management of Pregnancy Complicated by Diabetes*. Alexandria, VA, American Diabetes Association, 1993

Kitzmiller JL, Buchanan TA, Kjos S, Combs CA, Ratner RE. Preconception care of diabetes, congenital malformations, and spontaneous abortions. *Diabetes Care* 19:514–41, 1996

Langer O: Gestational diabetes: a contemporary management approach. *The Endocrinologist* 5:180–88, 1995

ASSESSMENT OF TREATMENT EFFICACY

In clinical practice, response to the treatment of type 2 diabetes mellitus should be monitored through a schedule of patient interviews and examinations with a comprehensive assessment of:

- continued patient acceptance of the treatment plan and goals
- symptoms
- weight
- blood pressure
- smoking
- screening evaluations for complications, including lipid levels and urine microalbumin
- various parameters of glycemic control

Among these parameters, glycemic control is unique in that techniques have been developed to allow both the patient and the health care team to independently and synergistically assess the response of glucose metabolism to therapy. This section will focus on assessment of treatment efficacy as reflected in glycemic targets (Table 3.15). In general, providers assess blood glucose control with assays for glycated hemoglobin. Intermittent measurements of fasting, preprandial, and postprandial plasma glucose levels in the office can also be useful.

For most patients, self-monitoring of blood glucose (SMBG) is critical in that it creates a situation in which the patients can be in control of their own therapy. If patients are aware of the glycemic targets associated with the outcomes they seek to achieve, SMBG provides a way for them to critically evaluate their response to therapy and to assure themselves that they are reaching their goals. In this process, it is essential that patients and practitioners agree on mutually acceptable glycemic targets, the frequency and pattern of SMBG, and a plan for interpreting and acting on the results obtained.

To this end, it is generally useful for patients to keep a daily diary of their SMBG results, not only so that they can periodically assess their results, but also so they can share them with the health care team. Sometimes recording food intake, activity, symptoms, and doses of diabetes medications simultaneously provides the patient and health care team with a better understanding of the factors that influence the level of glycemic control.

The frequency and type of monitoring of diabetes therapy should be determined in consultation with patients, taking into account the nature of their diabetes, their overall treatment plans and goals, and their abilities. A list of products available for SMBG and their features can be found in the American Diabetes Association's Buyer's Guide to Diabetes Products, an annual supplement found in the October issue of *Diabetes*

Table 3.15 Glycemic Control for People with Diabetes*

Biochemical Index	Nondiabetic	Goal	Additional Action Suggested
Preprandial glucose (mg/dl)†	<110	80–120	<80 >140
Bedtime glucose (mg/dl)†	<120	100–140	<100 >160
HbA$_{1c}$ (%)	<6	<7	>8

* The values shown in this table are by necessity generalized to the entire population of individuals with diabetes. Patients with comorbid diseases, the very young and older adults, and others with unusual conditions or circumstances may warrant different treatment goals. These values are for nonpregnant adults. "Additional action suggested" depends on individual patient circumstances. Such actions may include enhanced diabetes self-management education, comanagement with a diabetes team, referral to an endocrinologist, change in pharmacologic therapy, initiation of or increase in SMBG, or more frequent contact with the patient. HbA$_{1c}$ is referenced to a nondiabetic range of 4.0–6.0% (mean 5.0%, SD 0.5%).
†Measurement of capillary blood glucose.

Forecast. SMBG does require a modicum of manual dexterity, cooperation, and intelligence. With currently available equipment and established patient education techniques, there are few people who cannot successfully monitor blood glucose at home. The patient's socioeconomic circumstance is the critical issue for many, and too often determines whether SMBG is practical or not. Recent changes in federal and state insurance regulations are making SMBG a covered benefit for most insured patients.

Each of the assessment methods described below has advantages and disadvantages. Most often, a combination of methods is used to determine the degree of metabolic control.

OFFICE METHODS

When patients visit their health care providers, the clinician can assess the degree of blood glucose control with a laboratory plasma glucose determination, capillary blood glucose determination, and/or an assay for glycated hemoglobin. These measurements are of value in different ways. The plasma glucose or capillary blood glucose is an index of moment-to-moment control and can also be used to compare with simultaneously obtained patient SMBG results to check patient technique as well as the meter's accuracy. Glycated hemoglobin concentration reflects the level of glucose control for the preceding 2–3 mo and has been well established through the Diabetes Control and Complications Trial, as well as other prospective studies, to predict the risk of developing complications. Other glycated serum proteins can be measured in the laboratory. They reflect the level of glycemic control over shorter periods of time proportional to their circulating half-life.

Office Glucose Determinations

Fasting as well as 1- to 2-h postprandial glucose levels are easily measured and useful parameters for determining metabolic control. The major drawback to random plasma glucose determinations, particularly in a patient with moderate to severe disease, is that it is difficult to know what a single blood glucose determination reflects other than the level of glucose at that moment. Blood glucose levels can range widely during the day, so random determinations may represent peak values, trough values, or values in between. Furthermore, if the patient is visiting the office because of intercurrent illness, blood glucose levels will be of little value in determining overall glycemic control, as illness generally alters glucose tolerance. Also, some patients become more conscientious about following prescribed therapy just before office visits, in which case the random plasma glucose level may be misleadingly low. For these reasons, plasma or capillary blood glucose levels should be supplemented at regular intervals with an assay for glycated hemoglobin.

Glycated Hemoglobin Concentration

Glycated hemoglobin is expressed as a percentage of total hemoglobin, i.e., the fraction of total hemoglobin that has glucose attached. Depending on the assay method and laboratory used, the test may be called glycohemoglobin, glycated hemoglobin, glycosylated hemoglobin, hemoglobin A_1, or hemoglobin A_{1c} (HbA_{1c}). Although the different measurements all have different normal ranges, the results of all assay methods, when properly performed, correlate closely with each other. Efforts are underway to standardize these methods worldwide. Clinicians should become familiar with the assay used in their clinical laboratory, the factors that can interfere with it, and the normal range and should be vigilant for changes in the assay methodology used by the laboratories that they employ.

A glycated hemoglobin concentration may be used to assess the effects of changes in therapy made 4–12 wk earlier. It should not be used to determine the need for short-term changes in treatment. Blood glucose levels, generally from SMBG, are still the best means by which hour-to-hour and day-to-day changes in insulin management can be determined. However, health care providers have learned not to rely solely on SMBG results because the measurements are subject to errors in technique and the records are subject to errors of omission and commission.

Certain conditions and interfering substances affect glycohemoglobin results, depending on the assay method used. Any condition that increases erythrocyte turnover, e.g., bleeding, pregnancy, splenectomy, or hemolysis, will spuriously lower glycohemoglobin concentration in all assays. In addition, hemoglobinopathies, e.g., sickle cell trait or disease or hemoglobin C or D, will falsely lower glycohemoglobin results when hemoglobins are separated by nonspecific methods based on charge, solubility, and size. Other conditions, e.g., uremia, high concentrations of fetal hemoglobin (HbF), high aspirin doses (usually >10 g/day), or high concentrations of ethanol, may falsely increase glycohemoglobin levels. These artifacts do not occur in all methods, and specific reference to the manufacturer's package insert for the test assay used is the best guide to a particular assay's performance in various clinical situations.

Measurement of other glycated proteins, such as albumin or serum proteins, has been proposed as another means of determining average glucose control. These methods, including measurement of serum fructosamine, reflect a shorter period (~2–3 wk) of average glucose control than glycohemoglobin, as a result of the shorter half-life of serum proteins compared with hemoglobin. The shorter period of average glycemia reflected by the measurement of glycated serum proteins limits their overall utility similarly to the situation for single glucose determinations. It should be noted that it does provide theoretical advantages in situations in which the overall response to a recent (2–3 wk) change in therapy is necessary. However, although the glycohemoglobin assay does reflect glycemic control over a period of 2–3 mo, the result is time-weighted in that the level of glycemic control over the past month is a much greater determinant of the result than the previous months. Therefore, the glycohemoglobin test is fairly useful in assessing trends in response to therapy over a period as short as a month.

In general, well-controlled patients with type 2 diabetes and stable courses of treatment who perform home glucose monitoring should have their glycohemoglobin determined at least twice a year. More frequent monitoring of glycohemoglobin should be very useful in assessing the response to therapy in patients with unstable courses of treatment or changes in therapy, and in patients on insulin therapy or those failing to achieve glycemic control goals.

SELF-MONITORING

Between office visits, the patient can determine the degree of metabolic control by performing SMBG and keeping a record of test results.

Blood Glucose Monitoring

With the advent of SMBG and the availability of multiple pharmaceutical classes of drugs that attack the pathophysiology of diabetes in different areas, near-normal glucose levels have become a realistic goal for many patients with diabetes mellitus. Although in clinical trials SMBG has not been demonstrated to change outcomes in type 2 diabetes management when evaluated in isolation, many diabetes self-management training programs have been shown to help reduce complications (e.g., DIGAMI and Kumamoto studies). In all of these, SMBG was an integral part of the process, suggesting that SMBG is at least a component of effective therapy. Blood glucose monitoring is considerably more sensitive than urine glucose tests for the detection of hyperglycemia and provides the ability to detect hypoglycemia before it becomes symptomatic. SMBG, when combined with robust patient education, actively involves patients in the treatment process by allowing the patient to make adjustments in diet, exercise, and medication to achieve mutually agreed-upon targets. In the absence of periodic SMBG, it is almost impossible for patients to assess their response to the many activities that the health care team asks them to perform (e.g., nutritional changes, increased physical activity, and taking medications as prescribed). SMBG is an extraordinarily valuable tool in the education process to help ensure patient commitment to the therapeutic plan.

It is critical that patients have a well-established, concrete plan for action based on the results they obtain. Unfortunately, many patients faithfully perform frequent SMBG, record the results as instructed, and only discuss them with their health care team at semi-annual visits, despite the fact that their control is inadequate. Unless SMBG results are within agreed-upon targets, they should be communicated and reviewed at least monthly with a member of the health care team by phone, fax, mail, e-mail, or an interim visit to trigger changes in therapy as the need arises.

SMBG is particularly recommended for all patients on insulin or sulfonylureas, as it allows for the identification of minimal and/or asymptomatic episodes of hypoglycemia. It is well recognized that recurrent mild or asymptomatic hypoglycemia is a very strong risk factor for severe hypoglycemia. Although severe hypoglycemia is relatively rare in type 2 diabetes, it can have devastating consequences, such as trauma as a result of confusion or loss of consciousness. It is also commonly accepted that mild or unrecognized hypoglycemia is part of the reason why patients treated with insulin and a sulfonylurea have a proclivity for weight gain. Therefore, it is essential to have patients critically assess the nature of any "hypoglycemic" symptoms that occur during the day. Many patients are fearful or overconcerned about hypoglycemia and routinely consume extra calories when they are hungry, sweaty, nervous, or upset because they believe that they are hypo-glycemic. Monitoring generally documents that most symptoms in patients with type 2 diabetes are not related to hypoglycemia and should not be treated with food.

SMBG is also useful for patients with very early diabetes treated with lifestyle management (nutrition and activity), as it allows for day-to-day determination of the adequacy of their efforts. Furthermore, it gives patients the opportunity to assess glycemic excursions and contact the health care team early, if necessary, with deteriorations in glycemic control during periods of stress, such as those caused by infection or trauma.

Timing of SMBG will vary depending on the diabetes therapy. Useful times to monitor include before meals and bedtime (to assess the risk of hypoglycemia), 1–2 h after meals (to assess the maximal excursion in glucose during the day), in the middle of the sleep cycle (to assess whether there is any nocturnal hypoglycemia that can often be asymptomatic), and when experiencing symptoms (such as "hypoglycemic spells" or illness). It is important not to allow patients to get into the rut of only checking at one particular time of day. There are rare individuals in whom only a certain time of day is associated with abnormal results, and in those, more focused monitoring at that time of day may be appropriate. For some patients, their highest blood glucose of the day will be the morning glucose, and for others, their highest will be at another time of day.

Likewise, there are significant numbers of patients who have near-normal levels of premeal glucose who have substantial hyperglycemic responses to meals, particularly in the context of low-fat meal plans. Both in the setting of gestational diabetes and in well-controlled type 2 diabetes, 1-h postprandial capillary blood glucose levels have correlated more strongly with glycohemoglobin than fasting or premeal glucose levels. Patients with near-normal 1-h postprandial glucose levels clearly have excellent overall glucose control.

Some clinicians have patients concentrate on premeal glucose levels if the results are generally in the high 100s or higher. Once the premeal glucose levels reach the middle to low 100s, the patients switch to targeting 1- to 2-h postprandial glucose levels, as that amplifies the effects of lifestyle issues on glycemia and allows patients to identify how moderate changes in meal plan, activity, and medications have a significant impact on glycemic control. Even after substantial inappropriate changes in food intake, activity, or timing or dose of medication, blood glucose values often return to near-normal levels overnight or by the time the next meal comes around. Targeting therapy to SMBG results at just one time of day could leave the patient with a less than ideal overall response to therapy.

The frequency of SMBG needs to be matched to individual patient needs and treatment. Most clinicians ask patients on hypoglycemic agents to monitor at least once a day, varying before meals, bedtime, and mid-sleep, as well as when they have hypoglycemic symptoms. Some ask insulin-treated patients to monitor much more frequently (four or more times a day). In the subset of patients who achieve stable blood glucose levels, it is generally appropriate to decrease the frequency of SMBG to a few times a week, again generally concentrating on postprandial glucose levels. It is critical that SMBG be frequent enough that the patient and provider have a good understanding of both the adequacy of the treatment regimen and the stability of glycemic control.

There is now a wide assortment of meters available with many different features that may be very important to individual patients. The meters come in a wide variety of shapes and sizes, from the size of a pen to a card to a small box. Most have some memory for previous results, and some have sophisticated features that allow the user to record medication doses and symptoms. Use of meters that still require the strip to be wiped or blotted is not recommended, as that provides an extra step in which poor technique can affect results.

Some use significantly smaller sample volumes than others, which may be an advantage for patients who have difficulty obtaining an adequate drop. Similarly, some allow the user to wipe on blood and/or redose the strip if an inadequate volume of blood is applied to the strip initially. As a result, some meters are clearly much easier to use than others, especially for patients with a wide assortment of physical or cognitive impairments. Several can be adapted to voice synthesizers that provide audio output of results. The use of an automated lancing device for fingersticks is recommended. Several models are available: some more suited to children, those who frequently monitor, or the squeamish.

The bulk of the expense of SMBG is in the strips. It is generally possible for most patients to get a meter heavily discounted or for free. The role of the diabetes educator in helping patients determine which meter meets their needs and the role of vendors in minimizing the financial repercussions of SMBG are critical in making this technique as widely and appropriately applied as possible.

Urine Glucose Determinations

The determination of urine glucose has, for the most part, been superseded by SMBG. Urine glucose measurements are indirect and imprecise, and they should be reserved for patients who cannot or will not test blood glucose levels. The average renal threshold for glucose is ~180 mg/dl, but it can vary widely between patients and even in the same patient over time. A normal urine glucose cannot distinguish between hypoglycemia, euglycemia, or moderate hyperglycemia.

Urine Ketone Determinations

Patients with type 2 diabetes rarely have ketosis. However, some experts recommend home ketone testing in the presence of serious illness. Positive nonfasting urine ketones in a patient with type 2 diabetes is a worrisome finding that requires further evaluation.

Patient Records

The patient should be encouraged to keep a record of SMBG or urine glucose determinations in tabular form, so glycemic levels at various times of the day can be scanned visually with ease. Some meters contain memories that can be downloaded into a computer to produce such glucose logs. Generally, writing down glucose levels is still preferable because it allows patients to more frequently critically assess the pattern of glucose levels over time. On a long-term basis, the burden of keeping detailed logs of glucose monitoring, food intake, doses of diabetes medications, activity, symptoms (physical as well as emotional, including their circumstance and treatment), and the relative timing of all these parameters is generally more than most patients are willing to accept. Used intermittently, these kinds of records are invaluable in assessing how various lifestyle issues and therapeutic efforts interact in determining hour-to-hour and day-to-day changes in glycemic control. They are critical in developing lifestyle plans (diet and exercise) with patients and can serve to reinforce positive behaviors and to demonstrate their beneficial outcomes.

Patient records are also helpful to the health care team because they indicate the patient's degree of interest in control and provide information necessary for development of effective therapeutic plans. Almost all patients willing to keep records should be able to achieve excellent glycemic control, as they are clearly both willing and able to make substantial efforts in their self-care behavior. Furthermore, the records are usually invaluable in providing guidance about where to concentrate efforts in trying to improve glycemic control.

BIBLIOGRAPHY

American Diabetes Association: Self-monitoring of blood glucose (Consensus Statement). *Diabetes Care* 17:81–86, 1994

American Diabetes Association: Standards of care for patients with diabetes mellitus (Position Statement). *Diabetes Care* 21 (Suppl. 1):S23–31, 1998

Dagogo JS, Santiago JV: Pathophysiology of type 2 diabetes and modes of action of therapeutic interventions. *Arch Intern Med* 157:1802–17, 1997

deVeciana M, Major CA, Morgan MA, Asrat T, Toohey JS, Lien JM, Evans AT: Postprandial versus preprandial blood glucose monitoring in women with gestational diabetes mellitus requiring insulin therapy. *N Engl J Med* 333:1237–41, 1995

Faas A, Schellevis FG, van Eijk JTM: The efficacy of self-monitoring of blood glucose in NIDDM subjects: a criteria-based review of the literature. *Diabetes Care* 20:1482–86, 1997

Franz MJ: Lifestyle modifications for diabetes management. *Endocrinol Metab Clin North Am* 26:499–510, 1997

Goldstein DE, Little RR: Monitoring glycemia in diabetes: short-term assessment. *Endocrinol Metab Clin North Am* 26:475–86, 1997

Malmberg K, Ryden L, Efendic S, Herlitz J, Nicol P, Waldenstrom A, Wedel H, Welin L on Behalf of the DIGAMI Study Group: Randomized trial of insulin-glucose infusion followed by subcutaneous insulin treatment in diabetic patients with acute myocardial infarction (DIGAMI study): effects on mortality at 1 year. *J Am Coll Cardiol* 26:57–65, 1995

Ohkubo Y, Kishikawa H, Araki E, Isami S, Motoyoshi S, Kojima Y, Furuyoshi N, Shichiri M: Intensive insulin therapy prevents the progression of diabetic microvascular complications in Japanese patients with non-insulin-dependent diabetes mellitus: a randomized prospective 6-year study. *Diab Res Clin Prac* 28:103–17, 1995

Promoting Behavior Change

Highlights

Desirable Behaviors in Type 2 Diabetes
Healthy Eating
Regular Exercise
Appropriate Medication Regimen
Use of SMBG
Performance of Routine Foot Care
Proper Management of Illness
Development of a Support System and Coping Skills
Use of the Health Care System

Factors Influencing Behaviors

Techniques for Changing Behaviors
Assess Learning Needs
Identify Desired Behaviors and Goals
Plan and Set Goals and Objectives
Implement the Education
Documentation
Evaluation and Follow-up

Highlights
Promoting Behavior Change

■ Type 2 diabetes usually occurs in adulthood, a period of life when lifestyle patterns and behaviors have become firmly established. Optimal self-management of diabetes requires active participation by the patient in changing existing behaviors and adopting new behaviors. The entire health care team must assist the patient in behavior change. This process continues throughout life.

■ Success in achievement of behavior change involves education, skill development, and motivation of the patient regarding:

- healthy eating
- regular exercise
- taking diabetes medications safely, regularly, and at specific times

- performing self-monitoring of blood glucose and utilizing the information
- performing routine foot care
- properly managing illness
- developing a support system and coping skills
- using the health-care system

■ Individualized education and problem solving are at the heart of successful behavior change. The behavior change process is similar to the education process and involves assessment, planning, implementation, documentation, and evaluation.

Promoting Behavior Change

THE DIAGNOSIS OF TYPE 2 DIABETES generally occurs at a time in life when specific lifestyle patterns and behaviors have become firmly established. Optimal self-management of diabetes will require changing existing behaviors, as well as adopting new ones. A successful program for behavior change requires comprehensive patient education, skill development, and motivation. This is best accomplished through a team effort. Physicians, dietitians, nurses, and other health professionals, i.e., the health care team, should use their expertise to design a therapeutic regimen that promotes active patient participation in achieving the best metabolic control possible.

The importance of the health care team in managing diabetes was clearly illustrated in the Diabetes Control and Complications Trial (DCCT), where the level of desired glycemic control was accomplished only through the combined efforts of a treatment team. Not only did each member of the team actively participate in patient education and skill development, but each was able to provide regular and frequent follow-up, a crucial component of intensive management of diabetes.

It is during these ongoing follow-up encounters that the most active level of education and support in the behavior change process occurs. The knowledge and skills necessary to implement a treatment regimen cannot be acquired during a single encounter. Change occurs gradually over time and generally occurs in small increments. It is not uncommon for patients to experience periodic setbacks where motivation wanes and barriers to implementing behavior interfere with self-management of diabetes. At such times, the patient benefits from the experience and availability of the multidisciplinary health care team, which can provide not only specific problem-solving skills, but also necessary support. A health care system or environment must support these kinds of efforts if optimal diabetes control and subsequent improvements in patient health outcomes are to occur.

DESIRABLE BEHAVIORS IN TYPE 2 DIABETES

The goals of behavior change in type 2 diabetes are to adopt a healthy lifestyle and perform necessary diabetes management tasks. Although desirable behaviors may differ among individuals, they generally involve the following.

Healthy Eating

For most people with type 2 diabetes who are obese, modest calorie restriction and modification of eating behaviors to achieve and maintain even a minimal weight loss (10% of original weight) is an important behavior goal. All individuals with type 2 diabetes, regardless of weight, should benefit from following the USDA Food Guide Pyramid. The focus in these guidelines is to include a variety of foods and not encourage deprivation. (See the section on Nutrition in Chapter 3, Management.) The American Diabetes Association embraces these principles of healthy, realistic eating behaviors.

Regular Exercise

The benefits of exercise for people with type 2 diabetes make adoption of regular exercise a desirable behavior. Blood glucose control, blood lipids, and general fitness are improved with a regular exercise routine that occurs at least 3 times/wk. Obese individuals usually require exercise 5 times/wk to successfully lose weight. (See the section on Exercise in Chapter 3, Management.) Ideally, exercise should be both aerobic and strengthening. This may be difficult for someone who may have spent a lifetime avoiding physical activity.

Appropriate Medication Regimen

It's important for the person with diabetes to take diabetes medications safely, regularly, and at specific times. This may not be a problem for most individuals with type 2 diabetes, but it is sometimes for the elderly. Patients may forget whether they took their medication, take the wrong dose, or deliberately not take it because they think they don't need it. Some elderly people with type 2 diabetes may become confused because they take multiple medications.

Use of SMBG

Patients need to know how to perform self-monitoring of blood glucose (SMBG) and use the information to better manage their diabetes.

The discomfort and cost of performing SMBG is often a deterrent to patients with type 2 diabetes. This can limit the usefulness of SMBG in fine-tuning the diet or medication regimen. Clinicians need to make use of the SMBG data and teach patients how to use the information to alter nutrition, exercise, and medication. (See Self-Monitoring, p. 82).

Performance of Routine Foot Care

Older individuals are more susceptible to foot problems associated with diabetes and need to examine their feet routinely. Desired behaviors for proper foot care include smoking cessation, wearing well-fitted shoes, keeping feet clean, avoiding foot injury, and knowing what foot problems need medical attention.

Proper Management of Illness

Knowing how to maintain proper nutrition and hydration are important in managing illness in diabetes, particularly in older individuals. Knowing when to call a health care team member is important in maintaining independence, as well as in preventing serious complications.

Development of a Support System and Coping Skills

Stress may increase blood glucose levels. The management of diabetes coupled with the usual day-to-day hassles of life can be overwhelming. People with type 2 diabetes often have children, elderly family members, and demanding work schedules that leave little time for caring for personal emotional well-being. Having a support system makes the challenges of diabetes self-management easier to meet. Learning problem-solving skills, joining support groups, and educating family members about diabetes management are desirable behaviors.

Use of the Health Care System

Using the health care system includes keeping regular office appointments, following through with referrals to specialists, obtaining regular dental and eye examinations, and pursuing additional education as needed.

FACTORS INFLUENCING BEHAVIORS

Several factors influence the ability to change established behaviors. Age, socioeconomic status, and education level do not predict a patient's likeliness of adhering to a particular treatment regimen as much as complexity of the regimen and the relationship that is established between the patient and the health care team.

An individual's perception or belief regarding susceptibility to the consequences of diabetes can also influence his or her successful adoption of the new behavior. This health belief model suggests that a patient's perception of the benefits and barriers that result from taking action influence ability to change. Someone may, for example, feel that reducing fat intake to reduce cardiovascular risk is not necessary because he or she has had no problems and does not wish to give up high-fat foods.

The self-efficacy model suggests that, to make a behavior change, patients need to believe they have the ability to make the change with a reasonable amount of effort. For example, performing SMBG daily before breakfast and dinner may be possible, but doing it before lunch may not.

Specific patient coping skills may influence an individual's ability to change or learn new behaviors. A new diagnosis of diabetes may generate denial, anger, guilt, depression, and, ideally, acceptance. Such emotions can immobilize a person in his or her efforts to actively participate in self-management of diabetes. Often, fear brought about by lack of knowledge is an underlying cause of the inability to act.

The more complex a therapeutic regimen is, the more difficult it is to adopt (e.g., mixing insulins vs. premixed insulin preparations). The greater impact the regimen has on lifestyle, the more likely it is to be ignored (e.g., exercising daily given a demanding work or travel schedule). If negative consequences exist (e.g., sore fingertips with SMBG), the behavior will probably not be as readily adopted.

The relationship between the health care team and the patient affects behavior change. Patients and their health care teams who share a mutual respect for each other are more likely to be successful at achieving treatment goals. Mutual agreement on treatment goals and open communication regarding the barriers to achieving these goals are desirable behaviors.

TECHNIQUES FOR CHANGING BEHAVIORS

Despite the many behavior changes required in managing type 2 diabetes, most patients can become successful self-managers of diabetes. Clinicians need to be sensitive to factors that influence whether a patient is ready and willing to make changes and then devise a plan to facilitate the desired change. The process of changing behaviors can take many forms, but it generally occurs in a stepwise fashion (Table 4.1). Individualized education and problem solving are really the heart of successful behavior change. The behavior change process is similar to the education process and involves assessment, planning, implementation, documentation, and evaluation.

Table 4.1 Stepwise Behavior Change

- Assess learning needs and priorities
- Identify desired behaviors and goals
- Select behaviors to meet goals
- Obtain the knowledge and skills to implement behaviors
- Implement behavior change
- Evaluate the outcome
- Overcome barriers and select new behaviors

ASSESS LEARNING NEEDS

The first step in educating an individual to make behavior changes is assessment of knowledge, skills, and attitude. Current behaviors and lifestyle should also be thoroughly assessed. Generally, medical, lifestyle, and psychosocial data make up the assessment (Table 4.2).

IDENTIFY DESIRED BEHAVIORS AND GOALS

Based on assessment, currently performed desirable behaviors can be identified. Most patients are doing some things well and should receive

Table 4.2 Assessment Variables

- Demographics
  - age
  - occupation
  - insurance
  - economic considerations
- Medical history
  - vital signs
  - metabolic control values
  - general health
- Diabetes history
  - treatment regimen
  - duration
  - complications
  - diabetes education
- Nutrition habits
  - food preferences
  - eating patterns
  - caloric intake
  - supplements
- Physical activity
  - work activity
  - frequency and duration of other activity
- Lifestyle
  - sleeping habits
  - work
  - leisure time
- Psychosocial status
  - feelings regarding diabetes
  - family issues
  - stressors
- Educational factors
  - reading ability
  - visual acuity
  - dexterity
  - readiness

positive reinforcement for such behaviors. Desirable behaviors that need to be adopted can then become the focus. Providing the rationale for the desired changes helps the patient understand the importance of the behavior. Discussing realistic barriers to the performance of certain behaviors is important in setting behavior change goals with the patient.

PLAN AND SET GOALS AND OBJECTIVES

The patient needs to be actively involved in setting realistic goals and selecting behaviors they are willing to change. This allows the patient to prioritize what is most important to him or her at the present time. Setting goals first focuses efforts on a progressive accomplishment of behavior change. Selecting specific behaviors is the second part of this process. Behaviors should be specific and measurable, e.g., walking 5 min after breakfast on Monday, Wednesday, and Friday. Choosing goals and behaviors that are within reach builds on a patient's self-efficacy and promotes further success.

IMPLEMENT THE EDUCATION

Educating the patient by teaching necessary skills or providing the knowledge to perform the desired behavior in a format conducive to learning is critical to behavior change. The amount of information a person with diabetes eventually needs to learn is great. The National Standards for Diabetes Patient Education Programs specified 15 content areas. Actual content will vary with each individual based on his or her needs. Education can be survival level or be more advanced. Teaching problem-solving skills to overcome a barrier to behavior change is an example of more advanced education (e.g., how to find time to exercise as a single parent with small children).

Various teaching strategies can be employed (Table 4.3). With older adults, it is common that family members are taught in addition to the patient or instead of the patient. Involving family members in the education process will promote behavior change by enhancing the support network available.

DOCUMENT THE PROCESS

Because of the complex nature of instructions and the need to inform other members of the health care team, concise documentation of diabetes education is crucial. Appropriate problem solving through follow-up can only be accomplished with adequate documentation by health care team members. Documenting goals and instructions for the patient is also helpful. Writing things down assists patients in remembering instructions and priorities. This can be a valuable education tool.

Table 4.3   Teaching Strategies

- Methods
  - Individual instruction can be tailored to individual learning needs and focused on specific details of patient's self-management plan.
  - Group classes allow efficient use of educator time, and patients benefit from social support and peer learning.
  - Self-study is flexible, allows patients to pace learning; educator can monitor and evaluate progress.
- Techniques
  - Short lectures are effective for presenting new information.
  - Discussion allows patients to personalize information, ask questions, disclose feelings, and share experiences.
  - Skills training provides "hands on" learning; educator demonstrates, patient practices, then demonstrates, and receives feedback from educator.
  - Problem solving allows patients to integrate information on several topics, such as diet, insulin, and exercise, and to test their knowledge in hypothetical situations.
  - Role playing can be used to reinforce learning (patient plays educator role), to practice social skills (explaining diabetes to friends), and to explore personal problems (family stress).
  - Case studies provide an objective approach to learning that can be used for planning, problem solving, and to help patients identify errors they are making in their diabetes self-management.
  - Self-assessment methods, including blood glucose records, food diaries, and exercise logs, can be used to help patients recognize problems in their diabetes self-management, and often help to identify solutions.
- Materials
  - Printed materials can be used to reinforce teaching, for self-study, and as an information resource for future needs (e.g., sick-day guidelines).
  - Audio and visual aids, such as slides, films, overheads, audio and visual tapes, food models and labels, sample diabetes products, and dolls and puppets, are effective in enhancing learning.
  - Interactive learning programs available in printed, audio, visual, and computer formats allow individuals to learn at their own pace, with frequent evaluation to provide feedback on learning.
  - Games, such as crossword puzzles, board games, and group games, introduce fun into the educational process while enhancing participant learning.

EVALUATION AND FOLLOW-UP

Monitoring behaviors allows feedback regarding the success or failure of a particular approach to modifying that behavior (e.g., asking the patient to record how often he or she exercises). Linking behaviors to specific goals, such as changes in metabolic control, reinforces behaviors. For example, measuring blood glucose after exercise shows that exercise can reduce blood glucose levels. Involving the patient in the evaluation is essential. Evaluation is done after a specified amount of time has elapsed since the initial goal-setting session. Routine office visits or phone/fax contacts can serve as excellent follow-up evaluations. Patients can fax or phone in blood glucose results that can be discussed, and questions or problems can be identified and dealt with as they occur.

A crucial element in promoting behavior change is the problem-solving process. This is a skill that is best taught in follow-up sessions during those "teachable moments" when the patient perceives the need to learn and use the skills to solve a real problem.

BIBLIOGRAPHY

Peragallo-Dittko V, Ed. *A Core Curriculum for Diabetes Education.* Second ed. Chicago, IL, American Association of Diabetes Educators, 1993

American Diabetes Association: Standards of medical care for patients with diabetes mellitus (Position Statement). *Diabetes Care* 21 (Suppl. 1):S23–31, 1998

Haire-Joshu D, Houston C: Promoting behavior change: teaching/learning strategies. In *Management of Diabetes Mellitus: Perspectives of Care Across the Life Span.* Haire-Joshu D, Ed., St. Louis, MO, Mosby, 1992, pp. 565–92

Meeting the Standards: A Manual for Completing the American Diabetes Association Application for Recognition. Third ed. Alexandria, VA, American Diabetes Association, 1991

Non-Insulin-Dependent Diabetes: A Curriculum for Patients and Health Professionals. Ann Arbor, MI, Michigan Diabetes Research Training Center, 1993

Detection and Treatment of Complications

Highlights
Detection and Treatment
of Complications

■ Patients with diabetes are susceptible to numerous complications, both chronic and acute, as well as many adverse drug reactions.

■ The major risk factors for the macrovascular and microvascular complications of diabetes are:

- hypertension
- hyperlipidemia
- hyperglycemia
- lack of exercise
- smoking

Most of these risk factors are more prevalent in the type 2 diabetic population and act synergistically to promote vascular disease.

Major Chronic Complications

■ Men with diabetes are twice as likely and women with diabetes are 3–4 times as likely to die from coronary artery disease as men and women without diabetes. The average annual incidence of cardiovascular sequelae is increased at least twofold in patients with diabetes.

■ It is important to lower plasma lipid and glucose levels and to control hypertension, the latter being particularly important in terms of its benefits for reducing risks of microvascular (nephropathy and retinopathy) and macrovascular disease.

■ Hypertension is associated with an increased incidence and rate of progression of diabetic retinopathy and nephropathy and, therefore, must be treated aggressively. Potential complications with antihypertensive medications should be considered.

■ Nutrition planning and exercise programs should be used to help the patient achieve ideal weight and reduce dietary fat.

■ Cigarette smoking should cease.

■ Diabetic retinopathy does not cause visual symptoms until a fairly advanced stage has been reached, usually either macular edema or proliferative retinopathy. The changes involved in diabetic retinopathy may be subtle, which suggests that all patients with type 2 diabetes should have a complete evaluation at least once yearly, including visual history, visual acuity examination, and careful ophthalmoscopic examination with dilated pupils, by an eye doctor skilled in the examination of the retina.

■ A discussion of the clinical presentation of background and proliferative diabetic retinopathy is presented on pages 109–113. The indications for referral to an eye doctor are summarized in Table 5.4. Management of diabetic retinopathy is more successful when intervention is undertaken before visual symptoms develop. The ophthalmologic treatment of diabetic retinopathy depends on the stage of disease (page 112).

■ To monitor the onset of renal disease, a urinalysis (including microscopic analysis) and a serum creatinine should be done in all newly diagnosed patients beyond the age of puberty. Urinalysis should be repeated yearly in all adult patients.

■ Microalbuminuria usually is the first indication of renal disease and should be assessed yearly. Consultation with a specialist is suggested if persistent proteinuria, elevation in serum creatinine, or hypertension inadequately responsive to treatment is found.

■ More than 50% of the nontraumatic amputations in the United States occur in individuals with diabetes, and it has been estimated that more than half of these could have been prevented with proper care.

■ Early foot lesions often go undetected because they are usually painless. The prevention of foot problems requires proper foot care by the patient as well as early detection and prompt treatment of lesions by the physician. More serious foot problems are best handled in consultation with specialists in diabetic foot care.

■ The patient, with proper instruction, should assume major responsibility for prevention of foot problems. Minor noninfected wounds can be treated with nonirritating antiseptic solutions, daily dressing changes, and foot rest.

■ The diabetic neuropathies include the polyneuropathies of the upper and lower extremities and autonomic nervous system, lumbosacral plexus neuropathies, truncal radiculopathy, upper limb mononeuropathies, and cranial neuropathy. Neurotrophic foot ulcers are a complication of lower extremity polyneuropathy. The autonomic neuropathies include gastroparesis, diabetic diarrhea/constipation, neurogenic bladder, impaired cardiovascular reflexes, and impotence in men. Suggested approaches to diagnosis and management of these problems are presented on pages 118–122.

Major Acute Complications

■ The two metabolic problems of most concern in patients with type 2 diabetes are hyperosmolar hyperglycemic nonketotic syndrome and hypoglycemia in patients treated with insulin or sulfonylureas. Diabetic ketoacidosis may occur occasionally in patients with type 2 diabetes under severe stress (including severe infection).

■ The four major clinical features of hyperosmolar hyperglycemic nonketotic syndrome are:

- severe hyperglycemia
- absence of or slight ketosis
- plasma or serum hyperosmolality
- profound dehydration

■ Hypoglycemia can be precipitated by:

- decreased food intake
- intensive exercise
- alcohol and other drugs in combination with
- exogenous insulin
- sulfonylureas

■ Hypoglycemia should be suspected in a patient who presents with manifestations of altered mental and/or neurologic function as well as adrenergic responses. The diagnosis is confirmed by a plasma glucose level <60 mg/dl (<3.3 mmol/l).

■ If the patient is conscious, hypoglycemia should be treated by oral ingestion of some form of sugar. In the unconscious patient, parenteral glucagon or intravenous glucose may be necessary. Hypoglycemia may be prolonged in patients treated with sulfonylureas.

Detection and Treatment of Complications

MANY CLINICIANS consider type 2 diabetes mellitus a "mild" form of diabetes compared with type 1 diabetes because it characteristically has less labile glucose profiles and can often be managed satisfactorily with nutrition and exercise therapy or oral agents rather than with insulin. However, patients with type 2 diabetes are afflicted with the same litany of diabetes-specific long-term microvascular and neurologic complications as patients with type 1 diabetes (Table 5.1). Moreover, because type 2 diabetes generally affects an older population, it is accompanied by a high prevalence of premature cardiac, cerebral, and peripheral vascular disease, the risk of which is magnified two to sevenfold compared

---

Table 5.1   Chronic Complications Associated with Type 2 Diabetes Mellitus

Vascular Diseases

- Macrovascular
  - accelerated coronary atherosclerosis
  - accelerated cerebrovascular atherosclerosis
  - accelerated peripheral vascular disease

- Microvascular
  - retinopathy
  - nephropathy

Neuropathic Conditions

- Sensorimotor neuropathy
  - symmetrical, bilateral
    - lower extremities (most common)
    - upper extremities

- mononeuropathy
- neuropathic ulcer
- diabetic amyotrophy
- neuropathic cachexia

- Autonomic neuropathy
  - gastroparesis
  - diabetic diarrhea
  - neurogenic bladder
  - impotence in men
  - impaired cardiovascular reflexes

Mixed Vascular and Neuropathic Diseases

- Leg ulcers
- Foot ulcers

with the nondiabetic population. The occurrence of these complications, which can result in loss of vision, renal failure requiring dialysis or transplantation, amputations, heart attacks, strokes, and premature mortality, causes the greatest burden to patients with diabetes and belies the notion that type 2 diabetes is mild. Because type 2 diabetes accounts for >90% of diabetes in the United States, affecting over 15 million people, it contributes a major burden to health care. For example, type 2 diabetes is currently the single most common cause of new cases of end-stage renal disease.

This chapter reviews the detection, prevention, and treatment of long-term diabetes microvascular (retinopathy, nephropathy, and neuropathy) and macrovascular (coronary, cerebrovascular, and peripheral) complications that accompany type 2 diabetes. In addition, the acute metabolic complications of diabetes, including hyperosmolar hyperglycemic nonketotic syndrome and hypoglycemia and their management, are reviewed. Finally, patients with type 2 diabetes are often treated with numerous medications, including hypoglycemic, antihypertensive, and hypolipidemic drugs, to treat their diabetes and common coexistent disorders. The adverse effects of these medications and their interactions are also reviewed. Patient cases that illustrate proper diagnosis, prevention, and treatment of diabetic complications are presented on pages 124–131.

Prevention and treatment of the long-term complications of diabetes depend on reducing or eliminating identified risk factors for the development and/or progression of complications. Risk factors for the individual complications will be discussed in this chapter, and the benefits of risk-factor reduction will be presented. The Diabetes Control and Complications Trial (DCCT) demonstrated the benefit of good metabolic control in the development and progression of retinopathy, nephropathy, and neuropathy in type 1 diabetes. Although it was on a smaller scale, the Kumamoto Study confirmed that the beneficial effects found in the DCCT also apply to type 2 diabetes.

The risk-to-benefit ratio has not been examined for intensive therapy in type 2 diabetes and is of particular concern in elderly patients. The lack of studies defining the benefit of treatment in reducing macrovascular disease is a concern. Until such data become available, the risks and costs of therapy designed to achieve near-euglycemia must be balanced carefully against the putative benefits. Treatment should always be individualized, taking into consideration the patient's age and prognosis.

MAJOR CHRONIC COMPLICATIONS

ACCELERATED MACROVASCULAR DISEASE

In the patient with diabetes, atherosclerosis involving the coronary, cerebrovascular, and peripheral vessels occurs at an earlier age and with greater frequency than it does in people without diabetes and is responsible for 80% of the mortality in adults with diabetes. Thus, the clinician should be alert for signs and symptoms of accelerated atherosclerosis among patients with diabetes.

Early detection of complications is crucial so that appropriate treatment can be introduced before major morbidity or mortality occur. Although most patients with diabetes experience the same symptoms of coronary, cerebral, and peripheral vascular disease as patients without diabetes, clinicians should be aware that neuropathy and other factors may alter symptoms in the patient with diabetes. Patients with diabetes may have no or atypical anginal symptoms, such as exertional dyspnea, rather than exertional chest pain. In addition, cerebral manifestations of hypoglycemia may mimic transient ischemic attacks, and symptoms of neuropathy may need to be distinguished from symptoms of intermittent claudication.

Cardiovascular Complications

Studies have shown consistently that patients with diabetes mellitus have an excess of cardiovascular complications compared with patients without diabetes. In the United States, for example, those with diabetes are two-to-fourfold as likely as those without diabetes to die from coronary artery disease, and the average annual incidence of cardiovascular sequelae is increased at least twofold in patients with diabetes. Most important, the relative risk for cardiovascular disease in women with type 2 diabetes is 3–4 times greater than for women without diabetes.

Diabetes as a Cardiovascular Risk Factor

Type 2 diabetes is an independent risk factor for macrovascular disease. In addition, common coexistent conditions, including hypertension, dyslipidemia (decreased HDL cholesterol and increased triglyceride and LDL cholesterol concentrations), and obesity are also risk factors. The pattern of obesity is important, with central fat distribution (waist-to-hip ratio >0.9 in men and >0.75 in women) associated with dyslipidemia, hypertension, and increased prevalence of cardiovascular disease, independent of obesity. Other risk factors demonstrated in people without diabetes, such as smoking and lack of exercise, apply as well to people with type 2 diabetes. Finally, renal failure and even microalbuminuria may significantly contribute to the risk of macrovascular disease.

Importance of Modifying Vascular Risk Factors

Although most studies demonstrating the efficacy of reducing cardiovascular risk factors, such as hypertension and hyperlipidemia, in preventing or ameliorating cardiovascular disease have been performed in populations without diabetes, it is widely assumed that such interventions will similarly benefit those with type 2 diabetes. Indeed, subgroup analysis from several major trials supports this assumption. In the Scandinavian Survival Study (4S), the coronary heart disease (CHD) events were reduced in the subjects with diabetes, elevated LDL cholesterol, and prior clinical CHD in a similar fashion to the reduction found in the majority of subjects who did not have diabetes. Pravastatin therapy in the subjects with diabetes in the Cholesterol and Recurrent Events (CARE) study reduced new CHD events even when the baseline LDL cholesterol was not very elevated, much as it did in the subjects without diabetes. Therefore, clinicians should emphasize reducing these risk factors whenever possible.

Unfortunately, drugs used to modify some of the risk factors and complications in type 2 diabetes may worsen other coexistent conditions/risk factors. For example, antihypertensive treatment with thiazides in high doses or β-adrenergic blockers worsens atherogenic lipid profiles and glucose tolerance. Appropriate drug selection, such as cardioselective β-blockers and lower doses of thiazides, can usually avoid these problems, and these medications need not be avoided. Treatment of hyperlipidemia with nicotinic acid may also worsen glucose tolerance. Finally, more intensive efforts to lower hyperglycemia with sulfonylureas or insulin may increase obesity and hyperinsulinemia, although poor glycemic control is a greater detriment for the patient than these side effects. Clinicians must take care to select treatment regimens that do not worsen the overall risk for cardiovascular disease.

Hygienic measures, including weight reduction and exercise for obese patients with type 2 diabetes, are the most cost-effective and safe means of treatment and should be included in all treatment regimens. Successful weight reduction with a balanced diet will improve atherogenic lipid profiles, glucose intolerance, hypertension, and of course, obesity.

Low-dose (81–325 mg daily) aspirin has been demonstrated to be effective in reducing myocardial infarctions in subjects without diabetes in the Physician's Health Study and in multiple other studies. The Anti-Platelet Trialists reported a meta-analysis of 145 controlled trials of antiplatelet therapy. Both men and women with diabetes had a reduction in vascular events of a significant degree. The Early Treatment Diabetic Retinopathy Study (ETDRS) demonstrated the safety of aspirin therapy in people with diabetes and retinopathy and also found a reduction in myocardial infarction risk. As a result of these findings, the American Diabetes Association has recommended aspirin therapy in all people with diabetes who already have evidence of macrovascular disease and consideration of aspirin therapy in those at high risk because of family history, smoking, hypertension, albuminuria, obesity, and dylipidemia unless there is a contraindication. Enteric-coated aspirin in doses of 81–325 mg daily is recommended.

Hypertension. There is general agreement that control of hypertension reduces the development and progression of nephropathy and atherosclerosis. In addition, an association between retinopathy and hypertension has been documented in some, but not all, studies. Treatment of hypertension in patients with diabetes should be vigorous. The recent Sixth Report of the Joint National Committee on the Prevention, Detection, Evaluation, and Treatment of High Blood Pressure considered people with diabetes to be in the highest risk group, justifying early initiation of pharmacological therapy and a treatment goal of blood pressure <130/85 mmHg. Before initiating therapy, hypertension should be confirmed by repeat measurements. Automated ambulatory blood pressure monitoring may be especially helpful in people with diabetes who often lose nocturnal blood pressure reduction. Autonomic dysfunction and orthostatic hypotension should be excluded by measuring supine, sitting, and standing blood pressure.

The presence of diabetes may make the patient more susceptible to some side effects of drug therapy (Table 5.2). For this reason, there has

Table 5.2 Potential Complications of Antihypertensive Drug Classes in the Patient with Diabetes

Drug	Potential Complications
Diuretics	
Potassium-losing (thiazides, loop diuretics)	Hypokalemia, hyperglycemia, dyslipidemia, impotence
Potassium-sparing	Hyperkalemia, impotence, gynecomastia
Vasodilators	Exacerbation of CHD, fluid retention
Sympathetic inhibitors	Orthostatic hypotension, impotence, depression
Alpha-adrenergic blockers	Orthostatic hypotension
Beta-adrenergic blockers	
Nonselective	Cardiac failure, impaired insulin release with hyperglycemia, hypoglycemia unawareness, delayed recovery from hyperglycemia, impotence
Cardioselective	Blunted symptoms of hypoglycemia, hypertension associated with hypoglycemia, hyperlipidemia, impotence
Angiotensin-converting enzyme inhibitors	Proteinuria, hyperkalemia, leukopenia/agranulocytosis/cough

Cardioselectivity may be lost with high doses.
Adapted from Christlieb AR: Treating hypertension in the patient with diabetes. *Med Clin North Am* 66:1373-88, 1982

been disagreement regarding optimal drug therapy. Unfortunately, no large population-based randomized trials of the treatment of hypertension in people with diabetes have been reported. In spite of this deficiency, based upon more limited trials, some general recommendations for the treatment of hypertension in people with diabetes have emerged. Angiotensin-converting enzyme (ACE) inhibitors, α-blockers, calcium antagonists, or thiazide diuretics in low doses are preferred because they have fewer adverse effects on glucose homeostasis, lipids, and renal function.

ACE inhibitors have a particular attraction because they may have some unique renal protective effects of particular importance in people with diabetes. There is some caution necessary in the use of ACE inhibitors. Renal insufficiency may worsen in patients with bilateral renal artery stenosis, a problem that may be more common in type 2 diabetes. Diabetic nephropathy is associated with hyporeninemic hypoaldosteronism, and ACE inhibitors may cause unacceptable hyperkalemia in these patients. Angiotensin II receptor blockers may be substituted for an ACE inhibitor if unacceptable side effects occur, but more study is necessary to confirm their renal protective effects.

Peripheral α-blockers have no adverse effects specific to diabetes. Central sympatholytic agents may worsen orthostatic hypotension and sexual dysfunction. The studies on calcium antagonists have had divergent conclusions about their value in diabetes. There is some evidence that they have renal protective effects, particularly when combined with an ACE inhibitor. Other evidence suggests they have an adverse impact, particularly in comparison to ACE inhibitors.

In the past, the use of high-dose thiazide diuretics and β-blockers was controversial because these may increase cholesterol and triglyceride levels, lower HDL cholesterol, and exacerbate hyperglycemia. The adverse effects of thiazide diuretics are minimized when used in doses of 12.5–25.0 mg/day. Diuretics are very useful used in conjunction with ACE inhibitors. Caution is necessary when initiating ACE inhibitor therapy in patients on diuretics because hypotension may occur. Beta-blockers may have adverse effects on glucose and lipid metabolism and can interfere with hypoglycemia recognition and recovery. On the other hand, hypoglycemia is not usually a problem when treating type 2 diabetes, and β-blockers have been shown to reduce cardiovascular events in people with diabetes after myocardial infarction. The concern about the adverse effects of β-blockers in diabetes is outweighed by the benefits in these patients.

For patients with an isolated systolic hypertension >180 mm Hg, the goal is <160 mmHg. For those with systolic hypertension 160–179 mm Hg, the goal is a reduction of 20 mmHg. If these goals are achieved and well tolerated, further lowering to 140 mmHg may be appropriate. These goals may require use of more than one antihypertensive drug. The presence of autonomic neuropathy with postural hypotension may limit attempts to control blood pressure. Men with diabetes may be more prone to impotence as a side effect of certain antihypertensive drugs.

Lipids.   In type 2 diabetes, an increased prevalence of lipid abnormalities contributes to accelerated atherosclerosis. Characteristically, triglyceride-rich VLDL levels are elevated, and HDL cholesterol levels are decreased. LDL cholesterol levels are usually not different from those found in age- and sex-matched individuals without diabetes, but the LDL particles may be smaller and more dense, more oxidized, and glycated, all of which increases atherogenicity. Associated obesity aggravates the lipid abnormalities. This lipid profile is the result of a combination of altered synthesis, catabolism, and clearance. A fasting lipid profile is recommended at initial evaluation and yearly in people with type 2 diabetes.

The National Cholesterol Education Program (NCEP) recommendations for the screening and treatment of dyslipidemias are based predominantly on clinical studies in populations without diabetes. The American Diabetes Association has made some minor modifications to these recommendations specific for people with diabetes because of the high risk of atherosclerosis and the difference in the dyslipidemia commonly found.

- All patients with type 2 diabetes should be screened for dyslipidemia during their initial evaluation by measuring a fasting lipid profile, including triglycerides, total cholesterol, HDL cholesterol, and calculated LDL cholesterol.
- The increased relative risk for cardiovascular disease in women with type 2 diabetes and the common coexisting risk factors (e.g., hypertension) place the entire population with type 2 diabetes in a high-risk category.
- Medical nutrition therapy and increased physical activity are very important, particularly in reducing triglycerides and increasing HDL cholesterol. Either carbohydrates or monounsaturated fat can be increased to compensate for the reduction in saturated fat, but total fat must be reduced to reduce calories effectively.
- Side effects from nicotinic acid may have a greater impact in patients with diabetes, which should be taken into account when prescribing medications.

The most characteristic lipid abnormality in type 2 diabetes is an elevated triglyceride level and reduced HDL cholesterol. In many cases, elevated triglyceride levels can be satisfactorily lowered by improving glycemic control with nutrition therapy, exercise, oral agents, or insulin. Nutrition recommendations for these patients include a moderate increase in monounsaturated fat intake, with <10% of calories from saturated and polyunsaturated fats and a more moderate intake of carbohydrate. These recommendations might translate into a meal plan in which <30% of calories are from fat and 50–60% of calories are from carbohydrate. In patients with triglyceride levels >1,000 mg/dl, a reduction of all types of dietary fat to reduce levels of plasma dietary fat as chylomicrons is necessary. Acceptable borderline and high-risk lipid levels for adults are given in Table 5.3.

Patients without evidence of macrovascular disease in the borderline or high-risk category should be treated aggressively with diet, exercise, and glucose control. If these measures fail, the addition of LDL cholesterol-lowering drugs or triglyceride-lowering drugs, depending on the lipid profile, is indicated. Treatment of elevated LDL cholesterol is considered to have first priority. The LDL cholesterol level should be lowered to below 130 mg/dl in those without evidence of macrovascular disease and below 100 mg/dl in those with macrovascular disease. In high-risk patients, both nutrition therapy and pharmacological therapy may be instituted at the same time if the LDL cholesterol exceeds the goal by 25 mg/dl. Subgroup analysis of the subjects with diabetes in large trials of the HMG CoA-reductase inhibitors (statins) has shown the statins to be effective in reducing CHD. The statins are the most effective LDL cholesterol-lowering medications available, and they have an excellent safety profile. In high doses, some statins also reduce triglycerides significantly.

The bile-acid sequestrants, nicotinic acid, and gemfibrozil have also all been demonstrated to decrease cardiovascular morbidity in clinical trials that excluded or had very few patients with type 2 diabetes. In the Helsinki Heart Study, gemfibrozil treatment was associated with a non-statistically significant reduction in CHD in people with diabetes. In the absence of significant contraindications to their use, these drugs can also be used to treat hyperlipidemias in type 2 diabetes. At times, combination therapy is necessary. There is a low-level risk of significant myopathy when either gemfibrozil or nicotinic acid is used with a statin. Bile-acid sequestrants may increase triglycerides.

Data do not support a recommendation for a specific triglyceride level that will reduce atherogenic risk in type 2 diabetes. However, a

---

Table 5.3 Category of Risk Based on Lipoprotein Levels in Adults

	LDL Cholesterol	HDL Cholesterol	Triglyceride
Higher	≥130	<35	≥400
Borderline	100–129	35–45	200–399
Lower	<100	>45	<200

Data are given in milligrams per deciliter.

triglyceride level >1,000 mg/dl is considered a risk factor for pancreatitis and should be treated with medication. Treatment of lower triglyceride levels with medications is of unknown benefit. However, dependent on the clinician's judgment, when fasting triglyceride levels remain between 200 and 400 mg/dl despite dietary intervention and hypoglycemic therapy, lipid-lowering drugs should be used. Above 400 mg/dl, pharmacologic therapy is strongly recommended. In the presence of dyslipidemia characterized predominantly by elevated triglycerides, gemfibrozil is recommended. Nicotinic acid, although efficacious, may increase blood glucose levels and should be used cautiously.

Cigarette smoking.   Cigarette smoking is associated with accelerated macrovascular disease, and the presence of diabetes in a patient who smokes will further increase that individual's risk. Ongoing efforts should be made by the practitioner to assist the patient in discontinuing cigarette smoking, including enrollment in formal smoking cessation programs, behavioral modification, and use of nicotine patches.

Treatment of Macrovascular Disease

Clinical trials that examined the efficacy of secondary interventions (after clinical disease has occurred) have often excluded patients with diabetes. However, clinical experience and a limited number of trials in type 2 diabetes suggest similar efficacy of medical and surgical treatments of cardiac, cerebral, and peripheral vascular disease as that in nondiabetic populations, with several caveats. Anti-anginal treatment regimens and treatment of other risk factors after a myocardial infarction probably provide a similar benefit to both people with and people without diabetes. Clinical trials such as the Norwegian timolol study have included a sufficient number of patients with type 2 diabetes to demonstrate efficacy of β-blockade in preventing a second myocardial infarction. In insulin- or sulfonylurea-treated patients, the heightened risks of hypoglycemia with β-blockade must be taken into account. Vasodilators, ACE inhibitors, and calcium antagonists can generally be used safely in type 2 diabetes.

Despite the generally more diffuse coronary and peripheral artery disease in patients with type 2 diabetes compared with patients without diabetes, bypass surgery is an effective treatment, although patients do have an increased morbidity and mortality. The Bypass Angioplasty Revascularization Investigation (BARI) study did find that patients with multiple vessel disease had much better survival with coronary artery bypass grafting, including internal mammary artery grafting, than did patients undergoing angioplasty. It is not known if these findings apply to patients with more focal disease and the use of stents during angioplasty.

DIABETIC RETINOPATHY

The importance of frequent evaluation of and early detection and treatment of vision problems in patients with diabetes is illustrated by the following statistics:

- ~5,000 new cases of blindness related to diabetes are estimated to occur every year in the U.S., making diabetes a leading cause of new blindness among adults aged 20–74 yr.
- >60% of patients with type 2 diabetes have some degree of retinopathy 20 yr after diagnosis. At the same point nearly all patients with type 1 diabetes have retinopathy.
- Loss of vision associated with proliferative retinopathy and macular edema can be reduced by 50% with laser photocoagulation, if identified in a timely manner.

As in type 1 diabetes, the development and progression of retinopathy in type 2 diabetes is duration-dependent and associated with higher glycemic levels. Although more intensive efforts to control glycemia in the near-normal range in type 1 diabetes have been shown to definitely prevent or delay retinopathy, it is not known with the same degree of certainty whether a similar benefit will occur in type 2 diabetes. Attempts to normalize glucose levels, especially with low-risk treatments such as nutrition therapy and exercise, are appropriate. Although the role of hypertension in causing or accelerating diabetic retinopathy is less certain, control of hypertension is crucial to reducing risk for macrovascular disease and should be vigorously pursued. Relatively fewer patients with type 2 diabetes develop proliferative retinopathy than do those with type 1 diabetes; however, macular edema may be more common. In addition to retinopathy, patients with type 2 diabetes develop cataracts more frequently or at an earlier age than do people without diabetes.

Diabetic retinopathy does not cause visual symptoms until a fairly advanced stage has been reached, usually either macular edema or proliferative retinopathy. Management is more satisfactory when intervention is undertaken before visual symptoms develop. Therefore, yearly ophthalmoscopic examination by an ophthalmologist or optometrist who is experienced in diagnosing diabetic retinopathy is of crucial importance.

Types of Diabetic Retinopathy

There are three types of diabetic retinopathy: nonproliferative, severe nonproliferative, and proliferative.

Nonproliferative diabetic retinopathy (NPDR). The earliest stage of NPDR is characterized by microaneurysms and intraretinal "dot and blot" hemorrhages. NPDR occurs in most patients with long-term type 2 diabetes. In many cases, it does not progress and has no effect on visual acuity. However, if the abnormal vessels leak serous fluid in the area of the maculae (which is responsible for central vision), macular edema can occur with disruption of the usual transmission of light and a decrease in visual acuity. Macular edema may be mild and not immediately threaten vision or may be clinically significant macular edema (CSME) and require treatment because of the immediate threat to central vision. It is not possible for the general physician to be certain of the presence of macular edema with direct ophthalmoscopy. However, its presence can be suspected if there are hard exudates in close proximity to the maculae. Circinate hard exudates near the maculae are especially suspicious. Any of these findings should prompt referral to an ophthalmologist with expertise in diabetic retinopathy.

Severe NPDR.   Certain retinal lesions represent an advanced form of NPDR. When these lesions are found together, the risk of progression to the proliferative stage is increased. The severe NPDR lesions include cotton-wool spots (also referred to as soft exudates), which are ischemic infarcts in the inner retinal layers; "beading" of the retinal veins; and intraretinal microvascular abnormalities, which are dilated, tortuous retinal capillaries or, perhaps in some cases, newly formed vessels within the retina. When any of these severe NPDR signs are found, the patient should be referred to an ophthalmologist for further evaluation without delay.

Proliferative diabetic retinopathy (PDR).   The final and most vision-threatening stage of diabetic retinopathy is characterized by neovascularization on the surface of the retina, sometimes extending into the posterior vitreous. These vessels probably develop in response to ischemia. The prevalence of PDR among type 2 patients who have had diabetes for >20 yr may approach 30%. PDR poses a threat to vision because the new vessels are prone to bleed, especially if they are stretched by contraction of the vitreous. If bleeding into the preretinal space or vitreous occurs, the patient is likely to report "floaters" or "cobwebs" in the field of vision. The patient who has a major retinal hemorrhage will experience a sudden, painless loss of vision. The proliferation of fibrous tissue that often follows PDR can lead to retinal detachment as fibrous tissue contracts.

Prevention

The DCCT demonstrated that, in patients with type 1 diabetes, intensive treatment that lowers average glucose levels to near normal will prevent or ameliorate retinopathy. It is not unreasonable to assume that this finding also applies to the type 2 population. The small

Kumamoto study in Japan, conducted similarly to the DCCT, demonstrated benefit of improved control in type 2 patients, and the Wisconsin Epidemiologic Study of Diabetic Retinopathy (WESDR) found a strong association between baseline glycosylated hemoglobin and progression of retinopathy in type 2 patients independent of treatment. No other treatments to reduce the occurrence of retinopathy have been found. In addition, because photocoagulation decreases loss of vision by ~50% in patients with PDR or macular edema, identification of patients at risk in a timely manner is a major means of preventing loss of vision.

Evaluation and Referral

The changes involved in diabetic retinopathy may be subtle and escape detection by direct ophthalmoscopy. All patients with type 2 diabetes should have an annual examination with complete visual history, visual acuity examination, and careful ophthalmoscopic examination with a dilated pupil by an ophthalmologist or optometrist. The evaluations should begin from the time of diagnosis of type 2 diabetes, because the duration of hyperglycemia before diagnosis is uncertain and many patients will have established retinopathy at the time of diagnosis. The indications for referral are listed in Table 5.4. At this time, nondilated photographic retinal screening is available, but it is not considered a replacement for the annual examination because no rigorous studies have demonstrated equivalent diagnostic accuracy.

Table 5.4 Reasons to Refer Patients with Type 2 Diabetes Mellitus to an Ophthalmologist

- High-risk patients
  - neovascularization covering more than 1/3 of optic disk
  - vitreous or preretinal hemorrhage with any neovascularization, particularly on optic disk
  - macular edema

- Symptomatic patients
  - blurry vision persisting for >1–2 days when not associated with a change in blood glucose
  - sudden loss of vision in one or both eyes
  - black spots, cobwebs, or flashing lights in field of vision

- Asymptomatic patients
  - yearly examinations
  - hard exudates near macula
  - any preproliferative or proliferative characteristics
  - pregnancy

Note that visual acuity changes are frequently related to fluctuating glycemic levels and corresponding changes in hydration of the crystalline lens. Thus, a presenting symptom of diabetes in a patient may be a change in vision. Likewise, a patient whose glycemic levels are decreased in response to proper treatment may experience visual acuity changes and should be forewarned as well as reassured.

The multicenter Diabetic Retinopathy Study (DRS) and ETDRS defined three indications for immediate referral:

- vitreous or preretinal hemorrhage, even in the presence of normal vision
- neovascularization covering 1/3 or more of the optic disk
- macular edema

The risk of severe visual loss within 2 yr for patients with any high-risk characteristic is 25–50%, unless photocoagulation treatment is performed.

Treatment

The ophthalmologic treatment of diabetic retinopathy depends on the stage of disease. There is no commonly accepted therapy for non-proliferative retinopathy other than improved metabolic control. The ETDRS demonstrated that photocoagulation slowed progressive visual loss in patients with macular edema by 50%.

Panretinal photocoagulation is considered the treatment of choice for patients who have proliferative retinopathy with high-risk characteristics, and it reduces the risk of severe visual loss by about 60%. Photocoagulation is used to stop neovascularization before recurrent hemorrhages into the vitreous cause irreparable damage. Sometimes photocoagulation is used to treat eyes with PDR before high-risk characteristics have developed. However, the risks of photocoagulation are such that usually only one eye is treated; treatment of the other eye is deferred unless high-risk characteristics develop. When retinal detachment and massive vitreous hemorrhage occur, closed vitrectomy can be used to remove bloody vitreous and bands of fibrous tissue. During the procedure, clear fluid is infused to replace vitreous, and traction on the retina is relieved. In ~50–65% of cases, some sight can be restored with this procedure.

Patient Education

As the most important member of the treatment team, the patient must be fully informed about the possible visual complications of diabetes and their treatment.

- The newly diagnosed patient should be told that diabetic retinopathy, which can cause vision loss, is a possibility, and that it is important to report visual symptoms promptly.
- The patient should also be instructed regarding the relationship between hyperglycemia and diabetic retinopathy, with emphasis on the necessity to adhere to the prescribed treatment plan for diabetes.
- The patient also should know that hypertension may worsen diabetic retinopathy and that its diagnosis and treatment are important.
- The patient should know the importance of an annual dilated eye examination by an ophthalmologist or optometrist and that an examination for refraction may not be adequate.
- The patient should be informed of treatment possibilities (including photocoagulation) and the need for referral to an ophthalmologist familiar with the management of diabetic eye problems should serious retinopathy be detected.
- The patient with proliferative diabetic retinopathy should be informed that isometric exercises that raise intraocular pressure can aggravate proliferative retinopathy.
- The patient who is visually impaired or blind should be made aware of and referred to vocational rehabilitation programs and other social services.

DIABETIC RENAL DISEASE

The prevalence of diabetic renal disease is at least 5–10% 20 yr after diagnosis in patients whose diabetes was diagnosed after the age of 30 yr.

Clinical Presentation

The development of diabetic nephropathy is asymptomatic, and its detection relies on laboratory screening. The usual course of diabetic nephropathy in type 2 diabetes is not as stereotypical as in type 1 diabetes, but nephropathy tends to progress through a number of defined stages. The first sign of developing nephropathy is the occurrence of elevated microalbuminuria (>30 mg albumin/24 h). Whether microalbuminuria carries the same risk for the eventual development of clinical nephropathy in type 2 diabetes as it seems to in type 1 diabetes is unclear. As nephropathy progresses, "clinical" (dipstick positive, >300 mg albuminuria/24 h) proteinuria occurs, almost always concurrent with hypertension. Eventually, nephrotic range proteinuria develops, followed by decreasing glomerular filtration rate with rising serum creatinine until end-stage renal disease occurs.

Conditions That Influence Renal Function

In patients with diabetes, there are several conditions that either precipitate the development of nephropathy or exacerbate the condition when present.

Hypertension. Hypertension may precipitate the onset or further accelerate the process of renal insufficiency, or both. Virtually all patients with diabetes who develop nephropathy develop hypertension.

Neurogenic bladder. Neurogenic bladder may predispose the patient to acute urinary retention or to moderate and persistent obstructive nephropathy. In either case, renal failure may be accelerated.

Infection and urinary obstruction. When these occur together, the risk of pyelonephritis and papillary necrosis increases, and this may result in a decline of renal function. Repetitive urethral instrumentation increases the risk of urinary tract infections. Infarction of the renal medulla and papillae can occur from ischemic necrosis and infarction or obstruction and is typically accompanied by fever, flank pain, anuria, and accelerated loss of renal function.

Nephrotoxic drugs. Nonsteroidal anti-inflammatory drugs, chronic analgesic abuse, and contrast media radiographic studies have been associated with increased incidence and acceleration of renal failure in patients with diabetes. Nephrotoxic drugs should be avoided, and contrast media studies should be performed only after careful consideration of alternative procedures and with adequate hydration.

Prevention

To monitor the onset of signs of renal damage, a urinalysis (including microscopic analysis) and serum creatinine should be done in all newly diagnosed patients. A urinalysis and microalbuminuria determination if urine protein is negative should be done yearly in all patients. A 24-h urine specimen, overnight urine specimen, or timed urine specimen should be tested for microalbuminuria or the albumin:creatinine ratio determined on a random urine specimen. The finding of increased microalbuminuria or proteinuria should be followed by measurement of serum creatinine or urea nitrogen concentrations and assessment of glomerular filtration. If present, infection should be treated before the significance of the proteinuria can be determined.

The presence of microalbuminuria may be the first indication of advancing nephropathy and, if present, should prompt aggressive treatment of even modestly elevated blood pressure. To delay the onset and acceleration of renal disease in patients with diabetes, hypertension must be detected and treated aggressively. The ACE inhibitors are particularly beneficial in this regard. There are potential complications associated with the use of antihypertensive medications (Table 5.2), and these should be kept in mind when instituting therapy.

As with retinopathy, the DCCT demonstrated a decrease in development of microalbuminuria and clinical grade proteinuria with improved metabolic control. Although the evidence is less rigorous in type 2 diabetes, there is little reason to believe good glycemic control will not be beneficial. Consultation with a specialist is suggested if persistent proteinuria, an elevation in serum creatinine, or hypertension unresponsive to treatment is seen. Lower intake of dietary protein (~0.8 g per kg body wt per day or ~10% of daily calories) may have a role in reducing the rate of progression of nephropathy.

Patient Education

With regard to diabetic renal disease, the following patient education principles are suggested:

- Patients should know the importance of yearly urine tests.
- Patients should be told that the detection and treatment of hypertension is important because high blood pressure precipitates the onset of renal disease and accelerates its progression.
- Patients should be encouraged to have their blood pressure checked regularly and to adhere to therapy when prescribed. Patients should also be encouraged to limit their intake of dietary sodium and to achieve and maintain desirable body weight for the purpose of preventing or modifying the severity of hypertension.
- The symptoms of urinary tract infection should be explained, and the patient should be instructed to report such symptoms.
- Patients should know why the treatment of hypertension and recurrent urinary tract infection is important.
- The patient with signs of developing nephropathy should be told about the course of the disease and the options for treatment with dialysis and renal transplantation.

DIABETIC FOOT PROBLEMS

More than 50% of the nontraumatic amputations in the United States occur in individuals with diabetes, and it has been estimated that more than half of these amputations could have been prevented with proper care. Therefore, the clinician and patient who are conscientious about prevention, early detection, and prompt treatment of diabetic foot problems can make a significant impact on this problem.

Causes

Foot lesions in individuals with diabetes mellitus are the result of polyneuropathy, peripheral vascular disease, superimposed infection, or most often, a combination of these complications. Usually, foot lesions begin in feet that are insensitive, deformed, and/or ischemic. Such feet are susceptible to trauma, which may lead to callus formation, ulceration, infection, and gangrene.

In most patients with diabetes who have foot lesions, the primary pathophysiologic event is the development of an insensitive foot secondary to polyneuropathy. Loss of foot sensation is often, but not always, accompanied by decreased vibratory sense and loss of ankle deep tendon reflexes. Sometimes diabetic neuropathy is accompanied and worsened by other types of neuropathy, most commonly alcoholic or uremic peripheral neuropathy.

In addition to insensitivity, neuropathy may ultimately lead to a deformed foot secondary to tendon shortening (contractures), which leads to decreased mobility of the toes, abnormality in weight bearing, calluses, and development of classic "hammertoe" deformities. The combination of foot insensitivity and foot deformities that shift weight distribution promotes the development of foot ulcers. Neuropathy also causes decreased sweating and dry skin. If left untreated, cracked and thickened skin can lead to infections and ulcerations. Neuropathic ulcers in the patient with diabetes often go undetected because they are usually painless.

The sudden development of a painful distal foot lesion, usually secondary to trauma, may signify underlying peripheral vascular disease, which is associated with findings of decreased or absent pulses, dependent rubor, and pallor on elevation. The extent of the vascular disease and its potential for treatment by surgical intervention can be determined by Doppler noninvasive techniques and arteriography. Revascularization procedures, such as angioplasty and bypass, are often helpful in treating patients with severe disabling claudication (at rest) or nonhealing ulcers or to aid healing of an amputation incision. Unfortunately, surgical intervention is not always effective in individuals with diabetes because many may have diffuse vascular disease.

Infection is a frequent complication of both vascular and neuropathic ulcers. Studies indicate that these infections are often mixed and that gram-positive organisms predominate.

Prevention

The prevention of foot problems in a person with diabetes requires proper foot care by the patient as well as early detection and prompt treatment of lesions by the physician. Help from special health care professionals (podiatrist, orthopedist, vascular surgeon, and experts in shoe fitting) is frequently needed.

Physician responsibility. The first step in prevention is to educate all patients and to identify those who need a special or frequent evaluation because of risk factors for foot problems. During the evaluation, the examiner should determine whether the patient has experienced foot problems or intermittent claudication since the last visit. The physician also should conduct a thorough examination of both feet, looking for the signs and symptoms of impending foot problems (Table 5.5), which include foot deformities, calluses, and ulcers. The clinician should also check the pulses (dorsalis pedis, posterior, tibial, and femoral), search for bruits, and determine reflexes and sensation in the toes and feet.

Patient responsibility. The patient who has been given necessary information and proper instruction should assume major responsibility for prevention of foot problems. The patient (or family member, in the

Table 5.5 Warning Symptoms and Signs of Diabetic Foot Problems

	Symptoms	Signs
Vascular	Cold feet Intermittent claudication involving calf or foot Pain at rest, especially nocturnal, relieved by dependency	Absent pedal, popliteal, or femoral pulses Femoral bruits Dependent rubor, plantar pallor on elevation Prolonged capillary filling time (>3–4 sec) Decreased skin temperature
Neurologic	Sensory: burning, tingling, or crawling sensations; pain and hypersensitivity, cold feet Motor: weakness (foot drop) Autonomic: diminished sweating	Sensory: deficits (vibratory and proprioceptive, then pain and temperature perception), hyperesthesia Motor: diminished to absent deep tendon reflexes (Achilles, then patellar), weakness, sweating Autonomic: diminished to absent sweating
Musculoskeletal	Gradual change in foot shape, sudden painless change in foot shape, with swelling, without history or trauma	Cavus feet with claw toes Drop foot "Rocker-bottom" foot (Charcot's joint) Neuropathic arthropathy

(Continued)

Table 5.5 Warning Symptoms and Signs of Diabetic Foot Problems (*Continued*)

	Symptoms	Signs
Dermatologic	Exquisitely painful or painless wounds Slow-healing or nonhealing wounds or necrosis Skin color changes (cyanosis, redness) Chronic scaling, itching or dry feet Recurrent infections (e.g., paronychia, athlete's foot)	Skin: Abnormal dryness Chronic tinea infections Keratotic lesions with or without hemorrhage (plantar or digital) Trophic ulcer Hair: Diminished or absent Nails: Trophic changes Onychomycosis Sublingual ulceration or abscess Ingrown nales with paronychia

case of a patient who is impaired by morbid obesity or blindness) should be given instruction on how to cut toenails straight across and to inspect the feet daily for cuts, abrasions, and corns. The patient and family should know the importance of regular washing with warm water and mild soap followed by thorough drying. They should be instructed on the use of moistening agents, such as lanolin; the need to avoid prolonged soaking; strong chemicals, such as Epsom salts or iodine; and "home surgery." The potential hazards of heat, cold, new shoes, constricting or mended socks, and, especially, going barefoot should be emphasized to all patients, especially those with peripheral neuropathy.

Treatment

Minor noninfected wounds can be treated with nonirritating antiseptic solution, daily dressing changes, and foot rest. More serious problems, such as foot deformities, infected lesions, and osteomyelitis are best handled in consultation with specialists in diabetic foot care. Infected foot ulcers often require intravenous antibiotics, bed rest with foot elevation, and surgical debridement.

NEUROPATHIC CONDITIONS

The diabetic neuropathies are among the most common and perplexing complications of diabetes mellitus. Neuropathy has a wide variety of manifestations in people with diabetes, and the descriptive terminology and classification have also varied, causing some confusion among clinicians. A complete dissertation on neuropathy is beyond the scope of this chapter. Instead, a few important points about diagnosis and treatment of commonly encountered neuropathic problems are discussed.

Polyneuropathy

Polyneuropathy begins as a generalized, asymptomatic dysfunction of sensorimotor or autonomic peripheral nerve fibers. The sensorimotor neuropathy is symmetric and first involves the distal lower extremities. The presence and severity of the neuropathy generally relates to the duration of diabetes and degree of hyperglycemia. In people with type 2 diabetes, polyneuropathy may be present at the diagnosis of diabetes. In these cases, one assumes unrecognized diabetes was present for many years before the diagnosis. Polyneuropathy is often associated with retinopathy and nephropathy.

Several stages in the progression of polyneuropathy have been identified. The first abnormality is an asymptomatic change in nerve conduction or reduction of the heartbeat response to deep breathing or the Valsalva maneuver. To define neuropathy, the changes should be present in two or more nerves. Next, the patient is found to have decreased or absent ankle reflexes and/or abnormal vibratory sensation of the great toes. When present, symptoms can be either pain or relate to a loss of function. The pain intensity varies from causing discomfort to being disabling, and may be described as sticking, lacinating, prickling, burning, aching, boring, and/or excessively sensitive. Fortunately, most patients do not have pain and, when present, the pain may be a transitory phase.

Loss of pain does not necessarily imply improvement in the neuropathy. Functional loss is more common and is manifested by decreased tactile sense, lack of temperature discrimination, sensory loss, and muscle weakness. Inability to walk on the heels is a sign of more severe neuropathy. The muscular weakness may lead to foot deformity, such as hammertoes and abnormal weight bearing. The insensitivity leads to neglect of injury and contributes to foot ulcers (neurotrophic ulcers) and Charcot's joint.

Although polyneuropathy can affect the hands, most often hand symptoms are caused by carpal tunnel syndrome or ulnar neuropathy.

Autonomic Neuropathy

Diminished autonomic nerve function can cause an interesting variety of symptoms. Autonomic polyneuropathy, which usually occurs in concert with peripheral sensorimotor neuropathy, includes gastroparesis, diabetic diarrhea, neurogenic bladder, impaired cardiovascular reflexes, and impotence in men. Clinically, autonomic neuropathy tends to appear late in the course of diabetes.

Gastroparesis. The patient with gastroparesis may experience early satiety nausea, vomiting, and abdominal discomfort secondary to delayed emptying or retention of gastric contents. Other upper gastrointestinal abnormalities must be excluded before making a diagnosis of gastroparesis. Gastric emptying studies may be necessary to confirm the diagnosis. However, significant hyperglycemia can temporarily delay gastric emptying, so the glycemic control during the test should be monitored. Severe, symptomatic gastroparesis is uncommon in people with type 2 diabetes. Metoclopramide or cisapride is often helpful in treating gastroparesis. Erythromycin has been shown to improve gastric emptying and benefit some patients. Domperidone is an investigational drug that has been shown to be effective.

Diabetic diarrhea. Frequent passage of loose stools, particularly after meals and at night, marks the acute phase of this condition. Diabetic diarrhea tends to be intermittent and may alternate with constipation. Diphenoxylate (Lomotil), loperamide (Imodium), and clonidine have been shown to be effective to some degree. Some patients respond to treatment with a broad-spectrum antibiotic such as tetracycline.

Neurogenic bladder. Neurogenic bladder is characterized by a pattern of frequent, small voidings and incontinence and may progress to urinary retention. The demonstration of cystometric abnormalities and large residual urine volume are necessary for diagnosis. The patient with significant urinary retention may need to perform intermittent self-catheterization. Surgical intervention may rarely be required if the patient does not respond to conservative medical measures, because chronic urinary retention may lead to infection.

Impaired cardiovascular reflexes. Orthostatic hypotension and increased heart rates may occur when autonomic neuropathy affects the cardiovascular reflexes. Patients with orthostatic hypotension may find relief with the use of fludrocortisone and compression stockings. If fludrocortisone is prescribed, the initial dose should be 0.1 mg daily, and increases up to 1 mg should be made gradually. The drug should be used with particular caution in patients with cardiac disease, because it causes sodium and water retention and thus can precipitate congestive heart failure. Clonidine, a central alpha$_2$-receptor-blocking agent, has been used to treat this condition. Midodine is a newer agent that has been shown to benefit some patients.

Impotence in men. Impotence is a frequent occurrence in men with diabetes and usually manifests as lack of a firm, sustained erection. In most cases, libido and ejaculatory function are not affected, although retrograde ejaculation may be another feature of autonomic neuropathy. The measurement of nocturnal penile tumescence (NPT) is sometimes used to determine whether the patient's erections during sleep are normal, borderline, or abnormally diminished for age. When psychological and endocrine causes of impotence have been ruled out, the use of vacuum devices, intrapenile injections of vasodilating substances (papaverine, phentolamine, and prostaglandin), or intraurethral insertion of medication (alprostadil) allow the patient to resume sexual intercourse. The implantation of an inflatable or semirigid prosthesis is usually not required in the older patient with type 2 diabetes.

Other Varieties of Diabetic Neuropathy

In addition to symmetric polyneuropathy, people with diabetes are subject to a variety of other neuropathic syndromes that have no consistent terminology or classification applied to them in the medical literature. These syndromes include lumbosacral plexus neuropathies (also called femoral neuropathy or diabetic amyotrophy, depending on the clinical manifestations), truncal radiculopathy, upper limb mononeuropathies (the entrapment neuropathies—carpal tunnel syndrome and ulnar neuropathy, which are more common in people with diabetes), and cranial neuropathy. These varieties of neuropathy are asymmetric and abrupt or subacute in onset and tend to follow a monophasic course with improvement over time. They may be more common in type 2 diabetes, and their association with hyperglycemia is less clear-cut than that of polyneuropathy. In some cases, there is evidence that ischemia or inflammation is involved. Many patients have more than one type of diabetic neuropathy.

Lumbosacral plexus neuropathy may present with abrupt onset of asymmetric proximal muscle pain and weakness or, in its most severe form, with severe pain, wasting of the proximal muscles, and modest sensory involvement (diabetic amyotrophy). It is usually asymmetric and more common in men. Prominent features include quadriceps involvement, atrophy of thigh muscles, and absent patellar tendon reflexes. Complete recovery usually occurs in several months to a year.

Extraocular muscle motor paralysis, particularly that innervated by the third and sixth nerves, is the most noticeable of the cranial mononeuropathies. Patients can also develop peroneal (foot drop) and median or ulnar palsies. Spontaneous recovery in about 3–6 mo is usual.

Diagnosis

The diagnosis of a diabetic neuropathy is often easily made on clinical evaluation with little testing necessary. People with diabetes can have neuropathy unrelated to their diabetes. When the clinical features are not typical or consistent with the duration of diabetes and presence of other complications, other causes of neuropathy should be excluded.

Treatment

There is little evidence that any drug therapy is useful in preventing or curing diabetic neuropathy. The B vitamins have been used extensively but have not been proven effective. Treatment with tricyclic antidepressant medication such as amitriptyline (Elavil), or anti-epileptic medications such as carbamazepine (Tegretol) and gabapentin (Neurontin), may be helpful in some patients with painful neuropathy. A topical cream, capsaicin, is variably effective. Aldose reductase inhibitors have not been approved for therapy in the U.S., and the studies to date have generally been disappointing. Newer aldose reductase inhibitors appear to have greater promise. Aspirin, propoxyphene, and other analgesics should be prescribed as necessary for pain. Narcotics should be avoided, as the risk of addiction is high. However, sometimes narcotics may be the only effective method of pain control available. Physical therapy methods of treatment are often helpful.

MAJOR ACUTE COMPLICATIONS

The major acute complications of diabetes include metabolic problems and infection.

METABOLIC PROBLEMS

The two metabolic problems of most concern in patients with type 2 diabetes are hyperosmolar hyperglycemic nonketotic syndrome and hypoglycemia.

Hyperosmolar Hyperglycemic Nonketotic Syndrome

Of all diabetic comas, hyperosmolar hyperglycemic nonketotic syndrome is the most common in older patients with type 2 diabetes. When this condition occurs, it can be life-threatening. Hyperosmolar hyperglycemic nonketotic syndrome sometimes occurs in people with undiagnosed diabetes and in those with diagnosed diabetes after long periods of uncontrolled hyperglycemia.

Precipitating causes. There is almost always a precipitating factor (Table 5.6). Precipitating events include the use of drugs as well as other acute and chronic diseases (particularly infection) that increase glucose levels. Abnormal thirst sensation or limited access to water can also precipitate this syndrome.

Clinical presentation. There are four major clinical features of hyperosmolar hyperglycemic nonketotic syndrome:

- severe hyperglycemia (blood glucose >600 mg/dl [>33.3 mmol/l] and generally between 1,000 and 2,000 mg/dl [55.5–111.1 mmol/l])
- absence of or slight ketosis
- plasma or serum hyperosmolality (>340 mosM)
- profound dehydration

Typically, the patient develops excessive thirst, altered sensorium (coma or confusion), and physical signs of severe dehydration.

Treatment. The precipitating event should be determined and corrected as soon as possible while life-saving measures are employed immediately. Dehydration, hyperglycemia, electrolyte abnormalities, and the hyperosmolar condition should be corrected with use of appropriate fluids, insulin, and potassium.

Table 5.6 Factors Associated with Hyperosmolar Hyperglycemic Nonketotic Syndrome

Therapeutic Agents	Therapeutic Procedures	Chronic Diseases	Acute Situations
Glucocorticoids	Peritoneal dialysis	Renal disease	Infection
Diuretics	Hemodialysis Hyperosmolar alimentation	Heart disease Hypertension	Diabetic gangrene Urinary tract infection
Diphenylhydantoin	Surgical stress	Old Stroke Alcoholism	Septicemia Extensive burns
Alpha-andrenergic-blocking agents		Psychiatric Loss of thirst	Gastrointestinal hemorrhage
Diazoxide L-asparaginase			Cerebrovascular accident Myocardial infarction
Immunosuppressive agents			Pancreatitis

Adapted from Garcia de los Rio M: Nonketotic hyperosmolar coma. In *World Book of Diabetes Practice 1982.* Krall LP, Alberti KGMM, Eds. Amsterdam, Excerpta Med., p. 96–99; and Podolsky S: Hyperosmolar nonketotic coma. In *Diabetes Mellitus.* Vol. V. Rifkin H, Raskin P, Eds. Bowie, MD, Brady, 1981, Chapter 22.

Hypoglycemia

This metabolic problem occurs in patients with both type 1 and type 2 diabetes.

Precipitating causes. Hypoglycemia results when there is an imbalance between food intake and the appropriate dosage of drug therapy (i.e., sulfonylureas, insulin, or both). Exercise, intake of alcohol or other drugs, or decreased liver or kidney function can precipitate or exacerbate this imbalance.

Clinical presentation. Hypoglycemia should be suspected in a patient who presents with symptoms indicative of altered mental and/or neurologic function (changes in sensorium and behavior, coma, or seizure), as well as adrenergic responses (tachycardia, palpitations, increased sweating, and hunger). The diagnosis is confirmed if a plasma glucose level of <60 mg/dl (<3.3 mmol/l) is found when the patient is symptomatic.

Treatment. The objective of treatment is to restore the plasma glucose level to normal. When the patient remains conscious and cooperative, ingestion of some form of sugar by mouth (e.g., fruit juice, sugar cubes, glucose tablets, or a solution equivalent to 15–20 g carbohydrate) is usually followed by rapid relief of symptoms. In the unconscious or uncooperative patient, parenteral glucagon or intravenous glucose (50 cc 50% dextrose or glucose followed by 5% or 10% dextrose drip) should be given. In the setting of hypoglycemia secondary to sulfonylureas, hypoglycemia may be prolonged, and patients should be observed for at least 12–24 h.

INFECTION

The rapid diagnosis and treatment of infection in a patient with diabetes mellitus is absolutely necessary, because infection is a leading cause of metabolic abnormalities leading to diabetic coma. The more common infections seen in patients with diabetes mellitus and some critical comments about them are presented in Table 5.7.

PATIENT CASES

The following cases illustrate the most important points about diagnosis and management of the major complications of type 2 diabetes mellitus.

CASE 1: THE 51-YEAR-OLD EXECUTIVE SECRETARY

A.W., a 51-yr-old executive secretary with type 2 diabetes mellitus of 15 yr duration treated with nutrition therapy alone (although she had a course of treatment with glyburide for 6 yr until 5 yr ago), presents with a 3- to 4-mo history of progressive exertional dyspnea and easy fatigability. She reports no chest pain, except for an occasional episode of non-specific chest discomfort after sexual intercourse. She has not experienced nocturnal dyspnea, orthopnea, or peripheral edema. She reports a history of smoking one pack of cigarettes per day for 35 yr. Her family has no history of diabetes or cardiac disease.

Physical examination reveals an obese woman with a blood pressure of 138/85 mmHg, a pulse of 88 beats/min, and mild nonproliferative diabetic retinopathy. The cardiovascular examination shows a normal-sized heart without gallops or murmurs and good peripheral pulses without bruits.

Laboratory studies reveal a fasting plasma glucose level of 181 mg/dl (10.1 mmol/l), serum cholesterol of 245 mg/dl, triglycerides of 200 mg/dl, glycated hemoglobin of 10.1%, and serum creatinine of 1.1 mg/dl. The ECG and chest X-ray are unremarkable.

Because of the progressive nature of symptoms, an exercise thallium study is performed and shows an area of absent perfusion demonstrable only with exercise. The ECG abnormalities correspond to the anterior wall thallium defect.

The patient is treated with a course of β-blockers and calcium antagonists with elimination of her symptoms. A weight-loss program and low-fat diet coupled with a supervised exercise program result in weight loss, improvement of lipids, and normalization of the glycated hemoglobin.

Three years later, cardiac symptoms recur and do not respond to adjustment of medications. Coronary arteriography is recommended and performed. During the procedure, the patient is well hydrated, and a minimal amount of contrast media is employed. Proximal lesions are identified in two coronary vessels, with no distal lesions and good runoff.

The patient is referred for coronary artery bypass surgery. Six months after triple-bypass coronary artery surgery, the patient is symptom-free and stable.

Discussion Points

- Coronary artery disease is the leading cause of death in patients with type 2 diabetes, who have a two-to fivefold increased risk of coronary disease compared with the general population. The presentation is often atypical chest pain. Myocardial infarctions in patients with diabetes can be "silent" and occur without pain.
- Patients with diabetes often have involvement of more than one coronary artery. Contrary to popular myth, the lesions are often proximal and amenable to coronary bypass surgery. The 5-yr survival rates for patients with diabetes are improved substantially by surgical treatment.

Table 5.7 Infections That Are Common or Special to Patients with Diabetes Mellitus

Type of Infection	Comment
Cutaneous furunculosis and carbuncles	For reasons not clear, patients with diabetes mellitus may be prone to recurrent furunculosis and carbuncles. Unless vascular insufficiency is present, warm compresses may be used for treatment.
Vulvovaginitis (less frequently scrotal infections)	*Candida* skin infection commonly occurs in warm, moist areas, particularly in the region of the genitalia (also on the inner thighs and under the breasts). This is particularly common in people with type 2 diabetes who are overweight or who have been taking antibiotics. These infections can cause extreme discomfort to the patient and result in breakdown of skin, which may allow entry of more virulent organisms. Good glycemic control and local supportive antifungal treatment usually will resolve the problem.
Cellulitis, alone or in combination with lower extremity vascular ulcers	To prevent the spread of infection to bone and the necessity of amputation, treatment of infected ulcers and surrounding cellulitis must be aggressive. Antibiotics effective against bacteria recovered from the site (both aerobes and anaerobes should be expected), as well as surgical debridement and drainage, should be used.
Urinary tract	Asymptomatic bacteriuria occurs in up to 20% of patients with diabetes mellitus; some suggest that it be treated. Certainly a patient with neurogenic bladder is susceptible to urinary tract infection and sepsis. Treatment is mandatory in patients with pyelonephritis. Patients with serious urinary tract infections should be hospitalized, the offending pathogens identified, and appropriate susceptibility tests performed.
Ear	Malignant external otitis is relatively rare, but when it occurs, it is most often seen in elderly patients with chronically draining ear and sudden onset of severe pain. *Pseudomonas aeruginosa* is the usual pathogenic organism. This condition is fatal in ~50% of cases. Immediate treatment should include appropriate antibiotic therapy and surgical debridement when indicated.

Adapted from Rabinowitz SG: see Bibliography; and Casey JI: Host defense and infections in diabetes mellitus. In *Diabetes Mellitus: Therapy and Practice.* 3rd ed. Ellenberg M, Rifkin H, Eds. New Hyde Park, NY, Med. Exam., 1983, Chapter 32

- Because of the risk of contrast-media-induced acute renal failure, coronary arteriography should be performed under conditions of good hydration with a minimal amount of contrast material.
- Smoking markedly potentiates the risk of coronary artery disease, and patients should be advised to cease smoking.
- The hallmarks of diabetic hyperlipidemia are hypertriglyceridemia and lowered HDL cholesterol, which usually are proportional to the degree of hyperglycemia and are only partially responsive to glucose control.
- In patients with type 2 diabetes, hypercholesterolemia is common, usually mild, generally due to an increase of LDL cholesterol, and usually responsive to good nutrition management and regular exercise, including weight control, control of hyperglycemia, and reduction of cholesterol and saturated fat intake. Failure of the LDL cholesterol to fall below 100 mg/dl should lead to drug therapy.
- There is no evidence to suggest that patients with diabetes should be treated more or less aggressively with regard to surgical intervention. Medical treatment should be the first route, unless left main or left main equivalent coronary artery disease is suspected or present. Assessment of the efficacy of therapy may be problematic in many patients because of the lack of typical angina. Repeated exercise tolerance testing may be necessary to assess efficacy.
- Although the impact of risk factor reduction on preventing or delaying the need for bypass surgery is uncertain, the consensus is that vigorous efforts to lower cardiovascular risk factors are appropriate.

CASE 2: THE 48-YEAR-OLD ACCOUNTANT

C.B., a 48-yr-old African American accountant with type 2 diabetes of 10 yr duration treated with nutrition therapy and glipizide, presents for general medical care, having just moved into your community. His history is unremarkable except for some increased fatigability and nocturia.

Physical examination reveals a blood pressure of 185/105 mmHg, pulse of 84 beats/min, and fundi with some arteriolar narrowing, a few microaneurysms, and hard exudates. The patient has mild cardiomegaly with a prominent S4 but no murmurs. The remainder of the examination is within normal limits.

Laboratory studies show a fasting plasma glucose level of 205 mg/dl (11.4 mmol/l), glycated hemoglobin of 9.9%, urinalysis with trace proteinuria, and a serum creatinine of 1.9 mg/dl. The ECG reveals left ventricular hypertrophy, and the chest X ray shows an enlargement of the cardiac silhouette. Repeat blood pressure measurements on three other occasions are 190/105, 180/100, and 183/105 mmHg. There is no postural drop.

Treatment was initiated with atenolol. In response to progressively increasing doses, the blood pressure fell to 155/95 mmHg and the pulse to 55 beats/min. Prazosin was added, and the blood pressure fell to 145/90 mmHg. With the addition of clonidine, blood pressure was satisfactorily maintained in the range of 125–130/80–85 mmHg. Insulin therapy was instituted with morning NPH. Adjustment of the dose to 45 U lowered the glycated hemoglobin to 8%. With this treatment, the patient felt well.

Discussion Points

- Coexisting hypertension is of major concern in patients with type 2 diabetes mellitus because it increases the risks of atherosclerosis, renal disease, and proliferative diabetic retinopathy. It should be vigorously controlled, particularly in the presence of renal insufficiency, because adequate blood pressure control slows the rate of progression of nephropathy.
- The objective of blood pressure control should be to maintain the blood pressure as near to normal as possible (i.e., 120–130/80–85 mmHg) without postural hypotension.
- Diuretics are often used first in the treatment of hypertension. However, diuretic agents may impair endogenous insulin secretion and, thus, may exacerbate hyperglycemia in some patients. Diuretic use also may be associated with hemoconcentration, fluid and electrolyte imbalance, hyperuricemia, short-term dyslipidemia, and impotence. Diuretics in low doses may have minimal adverse effects while maintaining an effective antihypertensive action.
- Other antihypertensive agents that may be preferred for use in patients with diabetes include ACE inhibitors, calcium antagonists, and α-blockers. A cardioselective β-blocker drug (e.g., atenolol) or centrally acting drug (e.g., clonidine) may be used as second-line therapy. A cardioselective β-blocker does not impair glucose counterregulation unless used in large doses, at which it can also alter the patient's symptoms during hypoglycemia (i.e., decreasing trembling and tachycardia). Beta blockers may be less efficacious in African American patients. To promote patient compliance, the simplest possible dosage schedules should be used.
- Renal insufficiency in patients with type 2 diabetes (especially among African Americans) is a concern. Renal involvement generally begins 10–12 yr after diagnosis of diabetes. Annual urinalysis should be performed to detect renal involvement. If proteinuria is found, a serum creatinine or creatinine clearance should be obtained and the degree of proteinuria should

be measured. This patient might have done better with
an ACE inhibitor, considering his elevated creatinine
and proteinuria.

- In type 2 diabetes, the coexistence of hypertensive nephropathy is common. Treatment for diabetic and hypertensive nephropathy is similar. Lower intake of dietary protein (~0.8 g per kg body wt per day or ~10% of daily calories) may have a role in slowing the rate of progression of renal disease.

CASE 3: THE 56-YEAR-OLD LAWYER

P.L., a 56-yr-old lawyer with type 2 diabetes of 8 years duration treated with nutrition therapy and insulin, presents in your office for routine follow-up. When he undresses for his physical examination, he leaves his shoes and socks on. You ask him to remove them, and he replies that it is unnecessary to do so because his feet are fine. You insist.

Examination of his left foot reveals an ulcer 1.5 cm in diameter on the plantar surface over the first metatarsal head. Physical examination also reveals absent Achilles reflexes, decreased vibration sensation over the great toes and malleoli, and generalized sensory loss over the feet. Peripheral pulses are intact, and the feet are normal in temperature. Culture of the wound reveals mixed flora, and an X ray of the foot is unremarkable. The wound is cleaned, and the patient is fitted for a special boot to reduce weight bearing.

Discussion Points

- The feet should be examined frequently, especially in patients older than 40 and in those with a history of neuropathy, peripheral vascular disease, or foot deformities. Such evaluation should include a history of foot problems, paresthesias, or intermittent claudication; inspection of the feet, toes, and toe webs for ulcers, calluses, cleanliness, deformities, and fit of shoes; palpation of peripheral pulses (dorsalis pedis and posterior tibial); and determination of sensation and intactness of ankle reflexes.
- Patients should be taught proper foot care, including regular daily inspection of feet, cutting toenails straight across, not walking barefoot, washing feet regularly, using lanolin to prevent drying, breaking in new shoes slowly, avoiding heat or self-medication, and promptly seeking medical care for all foot lesions, including calluses.
- A warm, insensitive foot (i.e., neuropathic and pain insensitive) is at greater risk than a cool ischemic foot that feels pain.
- Once an ulcer appears in an insensitive foot, there should be absolutely no weight on the lesion. Antibiotics and debridement should be used as necessary.

- Peripheral vasculature can be evaluated by a Doppler stethoscope to determine the ankle/brachial blood pressure index (ABI); ABI values <0.9 signify the presence of vascular insufficiency.
- Patients with recently healed ulcers or with insensitive feet should try to decrease activities that increase barotrauma (pressure) on feet. Well-fitted orthotics (specially designed shoes) can help redistribute weight and decrease friction over pressure points, such as the metacarpal heads.
- Proper foot care is crucial in preventing recurrence of foot lesions.

CASE 4: THE 46-YEAR-OLD REGISTERED NURSE

H.M., a 46-yr-old registered nurse with type 2 diabetes of 9 years duration treated with nutrition therapy and metformin, presents for routine follow-up examination. Physical examination includes a funduscopic examination through dilated pupils. This reveals multiple microaneurysms, "dot and blot" hemorrhages, some hard exudates, and a few soft exudates. The patient is referred to an ophthalmologist.

Visual acuity is 20/20 in both eyes. The optic media are clear. Ophthalmoscopy confirms the presence of microaneurysms, dot and blot hemorrhages, and both hard and soft exudates. In addition, a few areas of venous dilation and some intraretinal microvascular abnormalities are noted. No maculopathy or neovascularization is seen. Photographs of the fundi confirm the above. A follow-up ophthalmologic appointment is arranged for 6 mo later.

Discussion Points

- Funduscopic examination is best carried out through dilated pupils by an ophthalmologist or optometrist experienced in the diagnosis and classification of diabetic retinopathy. Patients should be examined annually.
- Most patients with diabetic retinopathy, including proliferative retinopathy, experience no visual symptoms.
- Certain characteristics of diabetic retinopathy indicate a high risk for loss of vision, which can be lessened by treatment with photocoagulation. These high-risk characteristics are:
  - new vessels and preretinal or vitreous hemorrhage
  - new vessel on or within 1 disk diameter of the optic disk >1/4 to 1/3 the disk area in extent, even in the absence of preretinal or vitreous hemorrhage
  - macular edema

- The risk of blindness can be substantially reduced with careful and regular evaluations for early detection and with appropriate use of current therapeutic tools.

CASE 5: THE 58-YEAR-OLD CONTRACTOR

N.C., a 58-yr-old contractor with type 2 diabetes of 19 years duration treated with nutrition therapy and glyburide, presents for his annual physical examination. During the review of systems, he reports progressive erectile failure of ~1 yr duration. He says the problem began with inability to achieve vaginal penetration, and, most recently, inability to achieve any erection. Libido persists, but the patient is quite discouraged about his erectile incompetence. He reports no morning erections, does not use any medications except glyburide, and rarely consumes alcohol.

Physical examination is unremarkable except for decreased vibratory sensation in the lower extremities at the great toes and absent Achilles reflexes. The SMA12 is unremarkable except for a plasma glucose level of 174 mg/dl (9.7 mmol/l).

Urologic evaluation demonstrates normal genitalia but absent bulbocavernosus and bulbosphincteric reflexes. Serum testosterone and prolactin are normal. The urologist requests psychological consultation, including psychological testing. Results are normal.

The patient begins alprostadil urethral suppositories. Both he and his wife are satisfied with the results.

Discussion Points

- Psychogenic factors are the major cause of impotence in men without diabetes and should be considered in men with diabetes. Even when organic factors are present, many men have impotence due to a combination of psychogenic and organic factors.
- Neuropathic impotence in men with diabetes is usually associated with coexisting peripheral neuropathy. There is a higher incidence of neuropathic bladder changes in impotent men with diabetes. The bulbocavernosus and bulbosphincteric reflexes are often absent in men with neuropathic impotence. Vascular insufficiency has also been demonstrated in impotent men with diabetes.
- Neuropathic impotence is generally manifested by progressive erectile failure. Ejaculatory capacity usually is not affected.
- A variety of effective therapies are available, including vacuum devises, penile injections, urethral suppositories, and surgical implants.

BIBLIOGRAPHY

Abbott RD, Donahue RP, Kannel WB, Wilson PWF: The impact of diabetes on survival following myocardial infarction in men vs. women: the Framingham study. *JAMA* 260:3456–60, 1988

American Diabetes Association: Detection and management of lipid disorders in diabetes (Consensus Statement). *Diabetes Care* 16:828–34, 1993

American Diabetes Association: Management of dyslipidemia in adults with diabetes (Position Statement). *Diabetes Care* 21 (Suppl. 1):S36–39, 1998

American Diabetes Association: Standards of care for patients with diabetes mellitus (Position Statement). *Diabetes Care* 21 (Suppl. 1):S23–31, 1998

American Diabetes Association: Standards of medical care for patients with diabetes mellitus (Position Statement). *Diabetes Care* 17:616–24, 1994

The BARI Investigators: Influence of diabetes on 5-year mortality and morbidity in a randomized trial comparing CABG and PTCA in patients with multivessel disease. *Circulation* 96:1761–69, 1997

Bennett PH, Haffner S, Kasiske BL, Keane WF, Morgensen CE, Parving HH, Steffes MW, Striker GE: Diabetic renal disease recommendations—screening and management of microalbuminuria in patients with diabetes mellitus: recommendations to the Scientific Advisory Board of the National Kidney Foundation from an ad hoc committee of the Council on Diabetes Mellitus of the National Kidney Foundation. *Am J Kid Dis* 25:107–112, 1995

Colwell JA: Pharmacological strategies to prevent macrovascular disease in NIDDM. *Diabetes* 46 (Suppl. 2):S131–34, 1997

The DCCT Research Group: The effect of intensive treatment of diabetes on the development and progression of long-term complications in insulin-dependent diabetes mellitus. *N Engl J Med* 329:977–86, 1993

The Diabetic Retinopathy Study Research Group: Photocoagulation treatment of proliferative diabetes: clinical application of diabetic retinopathy study (DRS) findings. *Ophthalmology* 88:583–600, 1981

Gundersen T, Kjekskus J: Timolol treatment after myocardial infarction in diabetic patients. *Diabetes Care* 6:285–90, 1983

Kahn CR, Weir CG (Eds.): *Joslin's Diabetes Mellitus.* 13th ed. Philadelphia, PA, Lea & Febiger, 1994

Keen H, Jarrett J (Eds.): *Complications of Diabetes.* London, Arnold, 1982

Klein R, Klein BEK: Vision disorders in diabetes. In *Diabetes in America*, 2nd ed. Harris MI, Cowie CC, Stern MP, Boyko EJ, Reiber GE, Bennett PH, Eds. Washington, DC, U.S. Govt. Printing Office, 1995 (NIH publ. no. 95–1468), pp. 293–338

Klein R, Klein BEK, Moss SE, et al.: The Wisconsin Epidemiologic Study of Diabetic Retinopathy. III. Prevalence and risk of diabetic retinopathy when age of diagnosis is 30 or more years. *Arch Ophthalmol* 102:527–32, 1984

Klein R, Moss SE, Klein BEK: New management concepts for timely diagnosis of diabetic retinopathy treatable by photocoagulation. *Diabetes Care* 10:633–38, 1987

Levin ME, O'Neal W, Bowker JH (Eds.): *The Diabetic Foot.* 5th ed. St. Louis, MO, Mosby, 1993

Morgensen C: How to protect the kidney in diabetic patients. *Diabetes* 46 (Suppl. 2):S104–11, 1997

The National Diabetes Advisory Board: *The Prevention and Treatment of Five Complications of Diabetes: A Guide for Primary Care Practitioners.* Washington, DC, U.S. Department of Health and Human Services, 1983 (NIH publ. no. 838392)

Nathan DM: Long-term complications of diabetes mellitus. *N Engl J Med* 328:1676–85, 1993

Ohkubo Y, Kishikawa H, Araki E, Isami S, Motoyoshi S, Kojima Y, Furuyoshi N, Shichiri M: Intensive insulin therapy prevents the progression of diabetic microvascular complications in Japanese patients with non-insulin-dependent diabetes mellitus: a randomized prospective 6-year study. *Diab Res Clin Prac* 28:103–17, 1995

Orchard TJ, Strandness DE Jr: Assessment of peripheral vascular disease in diabetes. *Diabetes Care* 16:1199–1209, 1993

Physician's Health Study Research Group: Final report on the aspirin component of the ongoing Physician's Health Study. *N Engl J Med* 321:129–35, 1989

Rabinowitz SG: Infection in the diabetic patient. In *Diabetes Mellitus.* Vol. V. Rifkin H, Raskin P, Eds. Bowie, MD, Brady, 1981, Chapter 24

Rand LI: Retinopathy: what to look for. *Clin Diabetes* 1:14–18, 1983

Rosenstock J, Raskin P: Early diabetic nephropathy: assessment and potential therapeutic interventions. *Diabetes Care* 9:525–45, 1986

Scardina RJ: Diabetic foot problems: assessment and prevention. *Clin Diabetes* 1:1–7, 1983

Seltzer HS: Adverse drug interactions of clinical importance to diabetes. In *Diabetes Mellitus*. Vol. V. Rifkin H, Raskin P, Eds. Bowie, MD, Brady, 1981, Chapter 40

Singer DE, Nathan DM, Fogel HA, Schachert AP: Screening for diabetic retinopathy. *Ann Intern Med* 116:660–71, 1992

Joint National Committee: *The sixth report of the Joint National Committee on the prevention, detection, evaluation, and treatment of high blood pressure*. Washington, DC, U.S. Govt. Printing Office, Nov. 1997, (NIH publ. no. 98-4080)

Sowers JR, Epstein M: Diabetes mellitus and associated hypertension, vascular disease, and nephropathy. *Hypertension* 26:869–79, 1995

Vinik A, Milicevic Z: Recent advances in the diagnosis and treatment of diabetic neuropathy. *The Endocrinologist* 6:443–61, 1996

Index

Additional Resources from the Clinical Education Series

NEW!

Therapy for Diabetes Mellitus and Related Disorders, 3rd Edition

The "little green book" that guides thousands and thousands of healthcare professsionals worldwide through the treatment of specific patient problems has been completely revised and updated to meet ADA Clinical Practice Recommendations.

Representing the views and expertise of leading clinicians, each of its 54 chapters—many all new—focus on a different aspect of diabetes and present concise, practical approaches to treatment. Features new fast-acting insulins and oral drugs, including lispro, acarbose, troglitazone, and statins. Plus new recommendations for treatment of cardiovascular disease, impotence, foot ulcers, weight loss, and more.

Also included: Significance and Implications • Nutrition Management • Role of the Diabetes Educator • Metformin • Anti-hypertensive Therapy • Nephropathy • Noninvasive Cardiac Testing • Geriatric Patients • Ocular Complications • Alpha-Glucosidase Inhibitors • Dyslipidemia • Chronic Renal Failure • Insulin Allergy and Insulin Resistance • Much, Much More!

Softcover, about 400 pages, #5402-01
ADA member: $39.95   Nonmember: $49.95

NEW!

Medical Management of Type 1 Diabetes, 3rd Edition

Completely updated and revised to meet ADA Clinical Practice Recommendations. This new edition provides state-of-the-art instruction on all issues impacting patients with type 1 diabetes, including blood glucose regulation (featuring lispro, the new fast-acting insulin), nutrition, exercise, blood pressure, blood lipid levels, and more.

Also included: The Most Recent Changes in Diagnosis and Classification • Pathogenesis • Management of Objectives • Diabetes Education • Insulin Treatment • Monitoring • Nutrition • Exercise • Diabetic Ketoacidosis • Hypoglycemia • Pregnancy • Surgery • Maintaining Adherence • Developmental Considerations • Psychosocial Retinopathy • Nephropathy • Neuropathy • Macrovascular Complications • Limited Joint Mobility • Growth

Softcover, 224 pages, #5403-01
ADA member: $31.95   Nonmember: $39.95

NEW!
Intensive Diabetes Management, 2nd Edition

The ground-breaking, hands-on guide that delivers practical advice on achieving better blood glucose control through intensified management has been completely updated to meet ADA Clinical Practice Recommendations. Many key chapters have been revised to include specific instructions and various regimens for use of the new drug lispro with diabetic patients. You'll also learn why type 2 patients need to intensify their management and how to help them do it . . . why diabetes patients require continuing education and ongoing therapeutic adjustments . . . why achieving near-normal blood glucose should be done incrementally . . . how to tailor goals to an individual's needs . . . more.

Softcover, 192 pages, #5406-01
ADA Member: $31.95   Nonmember: $39.95

The Health Professional's Guide to Diabetes and Exercise

A practical, comprehensive guide to prescribing exercise as a therapy for diabetes patients. Examines the physiological aspects of exercise, as well as its metabolic and psychological benefits. Covers recommended forms of exercise; working with older patients, women, children, and patients with complications; advice for patients on insulin or other medications; nutritional concerns; much more.

Softcover, 352 pages, #5405-01
ADA member: $44.95   Nonmember: $49.95

Medical Management of Pregnancy Complicated by Diabetes, 2nd Edition

Incorporates the latest ADA Nutrition Recommendations. This valuable guide takes you through every aspect of pregnancy and diabetes, providing precise protocols for treatment. It's filled with techniques for managing blood glucose levels from the time of conception through every stage of pregnancy.

Softcover, 136 pages, #5401-01
ADA member: 34.95   Nonmember: $39.95

HOW TO ORDER

1. *To order by phone:* just call us toll-free at 1-800-232-6733 and have your credit card ready (Visa, Mastercard, American Express). Please mention code PK698IDM when ordering.
2. *To order by mail:* on a separate sheet of paper, write down the books you're ordering and calculate the total using the shipping and handling chart below. (NOTE: Virginia residents add 4.5% sales tax, Georgia residents add 7% sales tax.) Then include your check, made payable to the American Diabetes Association, with your order and mail to:

American Diabetes Association
ATTN: Order Fulfillment Department
P.O. Box 930850
Atlanta, GA 31193-0850

Purchase orders are accepted from recognized organizations for orders totaling $200.00 or more.

SHIPPING & HANDLING CHART

Up to $25   Add $4.99
$25.01–$60   Add $5.99
Above $60   Add 10%

Most orders are shipped with 72 hours of receipt. However, please allow 2–3 weeks for shipment. Add $4.99 shipping and handling for each extra shipping address. Add $15 for each overseas shipment. Prices and availability subject to change without notice.

About the
American Diabetes Association

The American Diabetes Association is the nation's leading voluntary health organization supporting diabetes research, information, and advocacy. Founded in 1940, the Association provides services to communities across the country. Its mission is to prevent and cure diabetes and to improve the lives of all people affected by diabetes.

For more than 50 years, the American Diabetes Association has been the leading publisher of comprehensive diabetes information for people with diabetes and the health care professionals who treat them. Its huge library of practical and authoritative books for people with diabetes covers every aspect of self care—cooking and nutrition, fitness, weight control, medications, complications, emotional issues, and general self care. The Association also publishes books and medical treatment guides for physicians and other health care professionals.

Membership in the Association is available to health care professionals and people with diabetes and includes subscriptions to one or more of the Association's periodicals. People with diabetes receive *Diabetes Forecast*, the nation's leading health and wellness magazine for people with diabetes. Health care professionals receive one or more of the Association's five scientific and medical journals.

For more information, please call toll-free:

Questions about diabetes:	1-800-DIABETES
Membership, people with diabetes:	1-800-806-7801
Membership, health professionals:	1-800-232-3472
Free catalog of ADA books:	1-800-232-6733
Visit us on the Web:	www.diabetes.org
Visit us at our Web bookstore:	www.merchant.diabetes.org